$8\underline{oc}$

DIMENSIONS
OF
NUTRITION

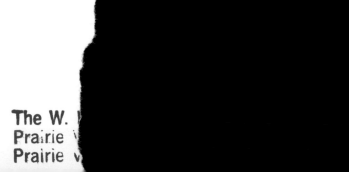

DIMENSIONS OF NUTRITION

Proceedings of a Conference Held
at Colorado State University
by the Colorado Dietetic Association
to Commemorate Its 40th Anniversary

EDITED BY

JACQUELINE DUPONT

COLORADO ASSOCIATED UNIVERSITY PRESS

Standard Book Number 87081-006-5

Library of Congress Catalog Card Number 71-134852

Copyright 1970 by Colorado Associated University Press

1424 15th Street

Boulder, Colorado 80302

TABLE OF CONTENTS

FOREWORD

To commemorate the Fortieth Anniversary of the Colorado Dietetic Association, a Conference "Dimensions of Nutrition" was held in July 1969. A group of outstanding speakers from a variety of disciplines assisted us to have an exciting and rewarding look at the many dimensions of nutrition.

This book reports the proceedings of the Conference. It is published to assist all those involved in the science of nutrition to develop a depth of understanding and an expansion of knowledge from the very basic level of metabolism to the application of nutrition principles. Forty years ago dietitians put vegetables in parchment bags and cooked them three times. They did not know why — or, as one dietitian stated, "I think it had something to do with harmful minerals." At this point in time we, the dietitians, nutritionists and other scientists, cannot afford to lack understanding in nutrition if we expect to take our place as specialists in the subject.

We are thankful to all who assisted us in the planning of the Conference. It is easy to have an idea, it takes much more effort to execute one.

Elisabeth P. Wirick
Conference Chairman and
President, Colorado Dietetic Association,
1968-69

CONFERENCE COMMITTEE

ELISABETH P. WIRICK, M.A., M.S., *General Chairman*
Associate Professor of Nutrition and Dietetics
Division of Nursing
Loretto Heights College, Denver, Colorado

JACQUELINE DUPONT, PH.D., *Program Chairman*
Associate Professor
Department of Food Science and Nutrition
Colorado State University, Fort Collins, Colorado

MARGARET M. BALL, M.S.
Assistant Professor of Dietetics in Nursing
University of Colorado School of Nursing, Denver, Colorado

VIRGINIA A. BEAL, M.P.H., NUTRITIONIST
Child Research Council
Assistant Clinical Professor of Pediatrics
University of Colorado School of Medicine, Denver, Colorado

JOAN E. CARTER, M.P.H.
Regional Nutrition Consultant
Health Services and Mental Health Administration
U.S. Department of Health, Education and Welfare

ESTHER M. EICHER, M.P.H.
Regional Nutrition Consultant
Children's Bureau
U.S. Department of Health, Education and Welfare

ACKNOWLEDGMENTS

The Colorado Dietetic Association extends thanks for contributions to this conference from:

ROCHE CHEMICAL DIVISION
Hoffman-La Roche Inc.
Nutley, New Jersey

DAIRY COUNCIL OF COLORADO, INC.
935 Eleventh Street
Denver, Colorado

THE COLORADO STATE UNIVERSITY
Fort Collins, Colorado

I

DIMENSIONS OF NUTRITION

DIMENSIONS OF NUTRITION

GRACE A. GOLDSMITH, M.D., Dean
School of Public Health and Tropical Medicine
Tulane University
New Orleans, Louisiana

The subject "dimensions of nutrition" could be discussed in at least two ways: 1) either the area or field of knowledge encompassed by the term nutrition could be described or 2) the impact of nutrition on society and its importance to the world of the future could be discussed. I will attempt to deal with this subject from both standpoints.

The science of nutrition covers a very broad area and many persons have had difficulty in delineating its boundaries. Nutrition is defined in the Encyclopedia Britannica as the science of food and the nutrients in food in relation to health. This is rather vague and non-specific. In 1963, the Council on Foods and Nutrition of the American Medical Association[1] proposed the following definition: "Nutrition is the science of food, the nutrients and others substances therein, their action, interaction and balance in relation to health and disease and the processes by which the organism ingests, digests, absorbs, transports, utilizes, and excretes food substances. In addition, nutrition must be concerned with certain social, economic, cultural and psychological implications of food and eating." This is a long and complicated statement but is much more specific and inclusive.

Recently, Sir Harold Himsworth,[2] former Deputy Chairman and Secretary of the Medical Research Council of Great Britain, gave an address at the dedication of the Dunn Nutritional Laboratory at Cambridge in which he suggested that nutrition was "the analysis of the effect of food- and its constituents on living organisms." He pointed out, relative to this definition of nutrition, that in the biomedical field we are dealing not with a subject but with a continuous spectrum of knowledge. "There is a single continuum from the specialized or mission-oriented research at the clinical extreme to research in unspecialized or basic biology at the other." In applying this concept to nutrition, he indicated that there is a range of research from the deficiency disease beriberi to the synthesis of thiamine, from rickets to the molecular significance of vitamin D, and from kwashiorkor to the intricacies of enzyme function. He further stated that in his opinion "the concept of natural intellectual continua of knowledge, stretching from specialized mission-oriented research at one extreme to unspecialized or basic research at the other, has genuine intellectual validity."

Such a concept enables dispensing with the categorization of research into fundamental and applied and substituting for this the more meaningful concept of specialized and unspecialized knowledge. It emphasizes that the flow of conceptual thought is not only from unspecialized or basic knowledge to specialized or mission-oriented, but also in the opposite direction. "It keeps in the forefront of our minds the thought that the survival of a subject as a separate intellectual entity depends not upon the basic discipline which is used, but upon the specialized investigations of natural experience from which it derives."

Himsworth went on to state that some persons have questioned whether the subject nutrition continues to exist and have pointed to activities that went on under the cloak of its name and asked if these differed from biochemistry. In disagreement with this philosophy, Himsworth illustrated nutrition research as follows: "the spectrum of knowledge was traced from the syndrome of beriberi down through the dietary defect that gave rise to it, through animal experimentation and the identification of the essential factor, to the final synthesis of thiamine." He suggested that this is an intellectual span that will bear comparison with any investigation in its grandeur.

Himsworth's definition of nutrition has been criticized by a number of persons as being too narrow. Several have pointed out that human nutrition is a problem of sociology, economics and politics as well as of science and technology. Keys[3] has agreed that nutrition is the study of the effects of food on living organisms and has opposed the view that nutrition is simply a special sector of metabolism which in turn is only a division of biochemistry. While the definition of nutrition as part of biochemistry is not far from the truth, Keys said, "I know what happens to nutrition when modern biochemists take over. Pretty soon the organism is replaced by isolated tissues and before long all attention is directed to events at the subcellular level. By all means let us applaud molecular biology but let us not forget that intact living people and even populations have nutritional problems that are too large to get onto the stage of a microscope."

Hegsted[4] also thinks that Himsworth's definition of nutrition is too narrow. He feels that nutritionists must be concerned with the entire process by which various kinds and amounts of food arrive in the stomachs not only of the physicians' patients but of all kinds of people: "It means concern with things such as agricultural policy, foods that are produced, processing which may enhance or detract from the food's nutritional value and make it more or less acceptable to the consumer, the distribution process which determines availability, and the cultural, educational, and financial factors which determine what is actually chosen and eaten. To limit our concern to the living organism eliminates from concern the important duties of dietitians and others involved in getting food to the patient and having it consumed." Hegsted quotes Commoner, who said, "The separation of the laws of nature among the different sciences is a human conceit. Nature is an integrated whole."

Some persons consider nutrition to be an ecological science. Certainly, nutrition is part of the environment and a most important one. Man in his domestication of animals and in the development of agricultural practices has upset many ecological systems, which is still another aspect of this whole science of nutrition.

This brief review of definitions will illustrate the wide scope of nutrition and, hopefully, will provide food for thought. No decision will be made as to a single, limiting definition or description of the science of nutrition.

Let us next discuss, more specifically, the dimensions of the science of nutrition in the year 1969 and the potentialities for the future. Professor Joshua Lederberg,[5] who received the Nobel prize in 1958 for his discoveries concerning genetic recombination and the organization of genetic apparatus of bacteria, presented the third Pan American Health Organization/World Health Organization lecture on the biomedical sciences. His subject was "Health in the World of Tomorrow." A number of his comments are pertinent to consideration of the dimensions of nutrition. He pointed out that the biological revolution of the last ten to twenty years was a philosophical one based on a new depth of scientific understanding about the nature of life. While there are still many mysteries of the detail about the way in which cells are constructed, no fundamental mysteries remain. It is feasible to think of creating a model of the cell and a model of life essentially on mechanistic terms. The essential substances that participate in the chain of life can be described. Most of the important gaps in our detailed understanding of the way in which the cell replicates have been filled in, e.g., the way it passes on information from generation to generation and the way it controls the synthesis of protein in its development. The cardinal element of this revolution is an understanding of the central significance of the role of DNA, of information transfer from DNA to RNA, and from RNA to protein. Life can be understood only in terms of these substances.

Lederberg went on to discuss the main health implication of the biological revolution which he considers to be "confidence in the eventual technical solubility of any biological problem now that we have passed the boundary of mysticism in our interpretation of biological processes. This was not true twenty years ago when we had only rather vague ideas about the chemical basis of heredity." He expressed confidence that problems such as that of aging can be solved and asked, "How are we going to cope with the inevitable success of our health research programs in fields like cancer, heart disease and aging in general?" He indicated that our preoccupation with the solution of these very urgent problems has made success seem almost out of the question. We must consider what success will mean to the nature of the population in which we live and to the nature of our own lives. "Will life be tolerable without death? Nothing more nor less than this is the inevitable fruit of our modern knowledge of molecular biology."

Lederberg made an interesting comment about malnutrition. He stated that it is a rather particular kind of genetic deficiency disease.

Man has evolved from precursors which had the capactiy to synthesize all the essential nutrients from rather simple sources in the diet. Now, man relies on plants which make all of the amino acids and vitamins. Man's requirements for specific food components can be stated as an evolved defect in his genetic apparatus. Whole sets of genes are lacking for the manufacture of tryptophan, lysine, threonine and so on. These genes are present in other organisms, for example, in many bacteria and most plants.

He suggested that it is plausible to foresee virological solutions to the problems of specific malnutrition that might be less expensive than maintaining an agriculture capable of producing an optimum variety of amino acids. He indicated that it will be necessary to learn how to graft viruses with genetic material of other origin and that such ability is not far away. Just one molecule of genetic information needed for the synthesis to tryptophan must be isolated from a cell of E.coli or a maize plant, for example. Then, a virus that carries the genetic information for the internal synthesis of tryptophan is introduced into a genetically deficient child (as all humans are) to produce this specific amino acid. Once this is done — and it could take place in the next few years — the international health experts will be asked whether it would be cheaper to vaccinate children against malnutrition than to teach them and their mothers how to maintain adequate and satisfactory diets.

In discussing the problem of the current rapid expansion of the world's population, Lederberg stated "by the same logic as we are dealing with malnutrition, we should also be able to produce a virus that will simply reduce the excessive fertility of the human species."

In the next few days of this conference on dimensions of nutrition, you will hear much more about nutrition at the molecular and subcellular level. Many recent investigations have dealt with nutrition and cell growth. Studies in this area indicate the important influence of nutrition on human growth and development. It is now possible, by chemical methods, to estimate the numbers of cells in an organ and the size of these cells. The amount of DNA in any organ reflects the number of cells within that organ, since the quantity of DNA is constant in the nucleus of all diploid cells of a given species. The total amount of DNA in an organ thus reflects cell number, and the weight of the organ as related to DNA, or the protein content of the organ as related to DNA reflects cell size.

Methods such as these have been applied in experimental animals and in man to determine the influence of malnutrition, particularly protein-calorie malnutrition, on brain growth and development at different time intervals.[6] Recent studies indicate that severe early malnutrition that leads to infantile marasmus and death in the first year of life results in marked curtailment of cell division in all organs including the brain. These infants have a reduction of from 20 percent to 60 percent of their expected number of brain cells.[7] The functional significance of this reduced cell number is not clear at the present time. As judged by animal experiments, this cellular deficit presumably will be irreversible unless rehabilitation is begun extremely early when cell division is still occurring. The fact that organs grow on a different time scale supports the concept of critical periods when nutritional interference in development may leave permanent defects.

Malnutrition in prenatal and early life is thought to affect subsequent mental development.[8] This is most difficult to prove scientifically as there are so many interrelated factors that influence development. It is hard to separate the effect of malnutrition from that of other environmental factors such as social stimulation. There is a known synergism between nutrition and infection and both of these factors have their roots in the social environment. Nutritional status is related to income, ethnic origin, occupation, habits, beliefs and taboos of a given culture. These findings indicate that studies of malnutrition in childhood reflect many of the dimensions of the science of nutrition from cell replication and organismal growth to ecology and the social structure of society.

At the other end of life, the role of nutrition in diseases which occur with aging again illustrates the dimensions of this science. Relationships between diet and serum lipid levels, atherosclerosis and coronary heart disease have been widely investigated. These investigations have included epidemiologic studies, basic studies of lipid metabolism and evaluation of various diets in the prevention and treatment of atherosclerosis and its complications. Additional studies are needed to understand the pathogenesis of atherosclerosis on a molecular and physiologic level, to learn more about arterial metabolism and the biochemistry of blood clotting, and to elucidate the role of nutrition in these processes.

As further illustrations of the broad dimensions of nutrition, scientists in this field continue to be interested in determination of requirements of essential nutrients under varying metabolic and environmental situations and elucidation of their specific roles in normal metabolism and in disease states. The importance of some of the minerals and trace elements, such as magnesium, zinc and chromium, are only beginning to be appreciated. These substances have an influence on numerous metabolic reactions and their significance in various pathologic processes affecting animals and man have become evident in recent years.

Interrclationshius among nutrients, and among nutrients and hormones, continues to be the object of considerable attention. The occurrence of naturally occurring toxic materials in food and the contamination of foods by substances such as aflatoxins or pesticides has been of great scientific interest. Another important area of study is that of interrelationships of drugs and nutrients. Some pharmacologic agents act as anti-metabolites and produce nutrient deficiency. Relationships between diet, the intestinal microflora and the nutrition of the whole organism continues to be a subject of study in both animals and man.

In recent years there has been a great deal of investigation of membrane structure and transport mechanisms as related to nutrition. These studies have been carried out at the molecular and subcellular level and also in vivo in animals and man. In human subjects, absorption of fats, protein, carbohydrates, vitamins and minerals has been investigated extensively under normal circumstances and in disease states. The effects of various dietary constituents on absorption are currently receiving attention, particularly as related to absorption of iron. Since iron deficiency anemia appears to be prevalent in the United States and in many other parts of the world today, this is of great public health importance.

Studies of genetic-nutritional interaction during development may have significance for many abnormal conditions in man other than those already known such as phenylketonuria and galactosemia. It has been demonstrated that interaction among genes and nutrients can result in a greatly increased requirement for a nutrient if deleterious effects of the gene are to be prevented.

Now, let us turn to the other aspect of the subject, dimensions of nutrition — namely, its impact on and importance to society and the world. It is obvious that adequate nutrition is essential for normal growth and development and for the maintenance of health of all forms of life. Nutrients are vital at the molecular, subcellular, cellular, organismal and human level and to the normal functioning of society as a whole.

Malnutrition is the most important public health problem in the world today and with each year it is likely to become more serious and extensive. The world's population is expanding more rapidly than at any time in history, particularly in the developing countries. As a result of dramatic declines in death rates without corresponding decreases in birth rates, the world population by the year 2000 may be double that of 1965, or six to seven billion people. To provide nutritionally adequate diets for this many more people will require much more food, especially more protein. The world food supply is not increasing at a rate proportional to that of the population expansion. To supply the world's food needs, there must be at least a 4 percent annual increase in food production over the next 25 to 30 years. This will be most difficult to attain, as in many areas the current rate of increase is in the neighborhood of 2 percent.

The world food problem[9] is one of tremendous dimensions and intricate, complex relationships involving more than public health, demography and family planning, and increased food production. It is fundamentally a social, economic and political problem, one of lagging economic development of the countries of Latin America, Asia and Africa, where two-thirds of the world's population now live. By the year 2000, there will be four times as many people in the developing countries as in the developed areas.

This is no time for us to become complacent in the United States. We have undernutrition and malnutrition here among us right now, in our society with its abundant food supply. The magnitude of the problem is not known, either in this country or elsewhere. The third World Food Survey of the Food and Agriculture Organization of the United Nations[10] suggested that at least 20 percent of the population in the less developed countries was undernourished, and 60 percent malnourished. In nutrition surveys in the United States,[11] findings thus far include undernutrition, obesity, goiter, iron deficiency anemia, and biochemical evidence of less than satisfactory nutritional status relative to a number of vitamins. The rates of growth of preschool children are considerably less than desirable.

The increased awareness of nutrition problems around the world has led to an increased interest in geographic pathology, in the refinement of diagnostic techniques for appraisal of nutritional status, and in the application of these techniques in order to learn the true extent and specific aspects of nutritional problems in many areas. Relationships between nutrition and agricultural development have received increased attention. The development of new and nutritionally more adequate sources of food has become a matter of high priority. The production of synthetic foods is being investigated. Policy-making agencies of government are devoting more attention to nutrition.

National and international groups, both public and private, must work together if the world food problem is to be solved. These dimensions of nutrition demand a global effort to grow more food and distribute it more equitably, to provide technical assistance for both agricultural and economic development, to assist in the education of professional and lay personnel in nutrition, to provide nutritional health services for those in need, and to develop programs to control the rapid expansion of the world's population. These are some of the dimensions and challenges of nutrition in the United States and in the world today.

REFERENCES

1. Council on Foods and Nutrition, Nutrition Teaching in Medical Schools, *Journal of the American Medical Association,* 183:995-997, March 16, 1963.

2. Himsworth, Sir Harold, What Nutrition Really Means, *Nutrition Today,* 3:18-20, Sept. 1968.

3. Keys, Ancel, Nutrition Definition, *Nutrition Today,* 4:1, Spring, 1969.

4. Hegsted, D. M., Nutrition Definition, *Nutrition Today*, 4:1 Spring, 1969.

5. Lederberg, Joshua, Health in the World of Tomorrow, *Third PAHO/WHO Lecture on Biomedical Sciences, Scientific Publication No. 175,* March, 1968.

6. Winick, M. and Nobel, A., Quantitative changes in DNA, RNA, and protein during prenatal and postnatal growth in the rat, *Dev. Biol.* 12:451, 1965.

7. Winick, M. and Rosso, P., Effects of severe early malfunction on cellular growth of human brain, *Pediat. Res.* 3:181-184, 1969.

8. Scrimshaw, N. S. and Gordon, J. E. (eds.), *Malnutrition, Learning and Behavior,* M.I.T. Press, Cambridge, Mass. 1968.

9. Panel on the World Food Supply, President's Scientific Advisory Committee: *The World Food Problem Vols. I and II,* Wash., D.C., U.S. Government Printing Office, May, 1967.

10. Food and Agriculture Organization of the United Nations, Third World Food Survey. *Freedom from Hunger Campaign, Basic Study No. 11,* 1963, p. 102.

11. Schaefer, Arnold E., in *Nutrition and Human Needs, Part 3.,* National Nutrition Survey, Wash., D.C., U.S. Government Printing Office, 1969.

II

NUTRITION AT MOLECULAR
AND SUBCELLULAR LEVELS

THE DEVELOPING NERVOUS SYSTEM

EFFECT OF PROTEIN DEFICIENCY IN THE RAT

ALAN B. GOODMAN, JON W. HARPER and JOHN R. BOLLES
Department of Physiology and Biophysics
Colorado State University
Fort Collins, Colorado

Introduction

Retarded physical growth during early childhood as a result of malnutrition is well documented.* The question has been raised, therefore, as to whether malnutrition, in particular protein malnutrition, affects the growth and development of the nervous system and thereby impairs learning and behavior.[1] The answer to this question is of interest not only to workers in the fields of nutrition, psychology, and neurobiology, but to all of mankind.

Research in this area to date has dealt only with the effect of protein malnutrition on the brain and has thus far ignored the rest of the nervous system. As a result the findings to be reviewed here are limited to the effect of protein malnutrition on the brain.

Cell Types in the Brain

The brain consists of two major cell types, neurons and neuroglia. One school of thought holds that both of these cell types develop from a common undifferentiated precursor, an indifferent cell.[2, 3, 4] This developmental scheme is shown in Figure 1.

---

*An excellent review of this problem is presented in *Malnutrition, Learning, and Behavior,* edited by Scrimshaw and Gordon, 1968 — the proceedings of an International Conference held at Massachusetts Institute of Technology in March of 1967.

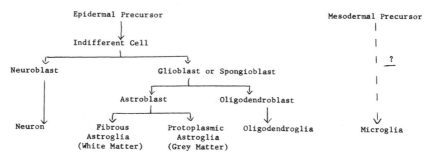

Fig. 1. A proposed developmental scheme for cells of the brain.

Mature neurons as seen in the visual cortex of rat brain (prepared with a modified rapid Golgi stain technique) are seen in Plate 1. Many dendritic processes arise from the cell bodies and show extensive branching. In addition, the proximal portion of the axon is visible at the mid-basilar aspect of the cell. The entire length of the axon is not visible due to the fact that this particular stain cannot penetrate the myelin sheath which surrounds the axon from this point on. Plate 2 shows a thin section (approximately 400 Å) through the cell body of such a neuron as seen with the electron microscope. This cell type can be identified as a neuron by several indicators:

1. a large and centrally located nucleus with typical chromatin dispersion
2. a large and centrally located nucleolus
3. a highly branched endoplasmic reticulum distributed throughout the cytoplasm
4. abundant polysomes and some free ribosomes
5. several perinuclear Golgi zones — usually 3 to 4
6. mitochondria with typical septate cristae (few exceptions)
7. occasional lysosomes and multivesicular bodies
8. axo-somatic synapses

Until recent years it was generally acknowledged that all neurons are formed prenatally and that a complete set of neurons is present at the time of birth. Recent studies, however, indicate that this is not the case. In the rat, for instance, a portion of neuron formation may take place after birth and, indeed, seems to depend upon adequate environmental stimulation for completion.[5, 6]

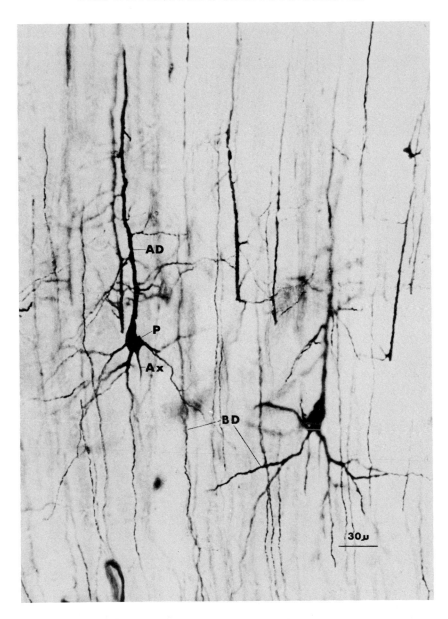

Plate 1. A modified Golgi preparation of the striate cortex of an adult rat showing the arborization characteristics of fifth layer pyramidal neurons. The background opacity, typical of all Golgi-type techniques, is delegated to the section by its extreme thickness, some 220 microns. P, perikaryon; AD, apical dendrite; Ax, axon; BD, basal dendrites.

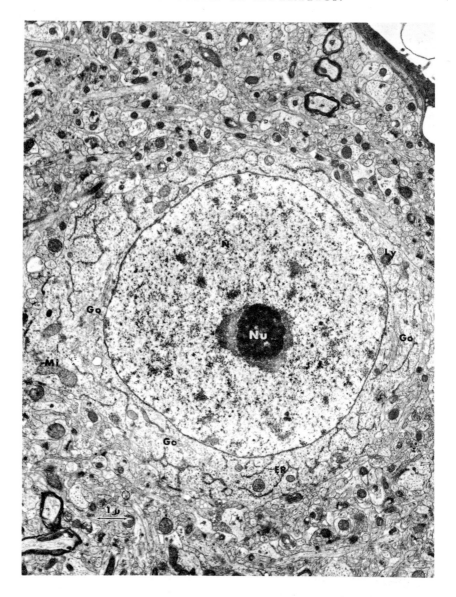

Plate 2. A typical neuron from adult rat visual cortex which is easily
differentiated from surrounding neuropil by its light cytoplasm, highly
branched endoplasmic reticulum (ER), numerous mitochondria (Mi), three or
four perinuclear golgi zones (Go), an occasional lysosome (Ly) and a
large, centrally located nucleolus (Nu). Magnification, 10,400X.

The neuroglia or glial cells constitute a large percentage of the total brain volume and are of two major types, the astroglia and the oligodendroglia. Plate 3 is an electron micrograph of an astrocyte which can be identified by the following features:

1. a clear and watery cytoplasm and nucleoplasm
2. a large and irregular nucleus with an occasional nucleolus
3. scanty organelles
4. large open vacuoles
5. glycogen granuoles
6. bundles of 60 Å filaments

These cells form a barrier between other brain cells and the blood vessels of the brain, the so-called blood-brain barrier.

The other major glial cell type, the oligodendroglia, is depicted in Plate 4. These cells do not contain the cytoplasmic filament bundles as do the astroglia, but, are characterized by:

1. large quantities of cytoplasmic ribosomes — indicative of a high rate of protein synthesis
2. more well-developed organelles
3. a regular ovoid nucleus with characteristic chromatin dispersion.

Oligodendroglia are in intimate contact with the cell bodies and all processes of neurons and appear to be responsible for myelinization in the brain. The proliferation of this cell type may also be dependent on the postnatal environment.[7, 8]

The extensions of both types of neuroglia are interspersed among adjacent neurons providing, among other things, nourishment and cytoarchitectural support of the neuronal population. The processes of glial cells may surround synaptic regions but are never found between pre- and post-synaptic elements.[9]

For several decades a third type of glial cell, the microglia, was thought to exist. Recently, however, several investigators, utilizing electron microscopic analysis, have come to question the actual existence of microglia, and it has been concluded that their presence in the brain must remain an open question.[10, 11]

The ratio of glial cells to neurons varies widely in different areas of the brain. Glial to neuron ratios of less than 1.0 to 10.0 have been reported.[8, 12, 13]

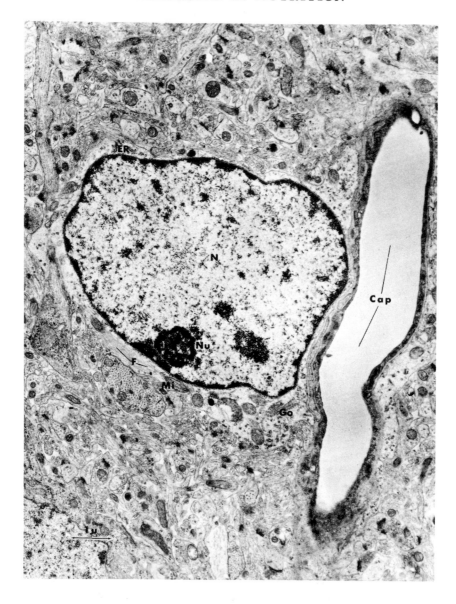

Plate 3. An astroglial cell from adult rat neocortex demonstrating the intimate astroglial-capillary relationship. N, nucleus; Nu, nucleolus; ER, endoplasmic reticulum; Go, golgi apparatus; Mi, mitochondria; F, 60 Å thick filaments. Magnification, 10,600X.

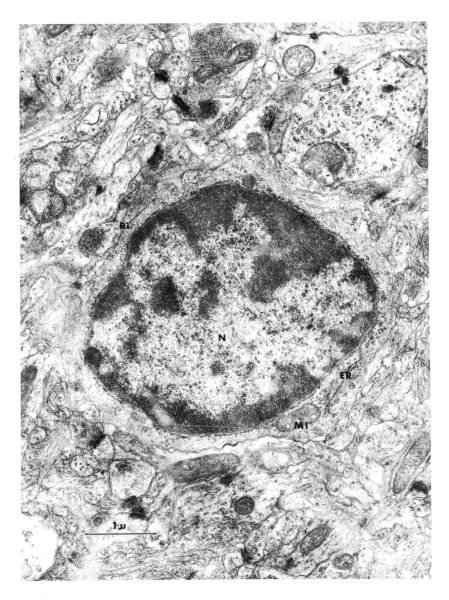

Plate 4. An oligodendroglial cell from the visual cortex of an adult rat. The cytoplasmic density is contributed in part by a large resident population of free ribosomes and polyribosomal profiles. N, nucleus; ER, endoplasmic reticulum; Mi, mitochondria; Ri, ribosomes (ribonucleoprotein granules). Magnification, 28,200X.

The Normal Development of the Brain

In general, the sequence of development of all mammalian brains is similar. Neuroblasts appear first, and the majority of the adult neurons are formed. There then follows a large proliferation of glial cells which is followed in turn by the manufacture of myelin sheaths by the oligodendroglia. The majority of brain growth always precedes the major growth of the body. Figure 2 shows curves depicting the rate of brain growth relative to the time of birth in several different species. Note that the rapid period of brain growth may be pre- or postnatal depending on the species investigated. It is important to keep this fact in mind as malnutrition will have to be instituted at distinctly different times in relation to birth in different species if the same developmental processes are to be affected. Note in particular the rat, since most of the evidence that has accumulated has been derived from this speies.

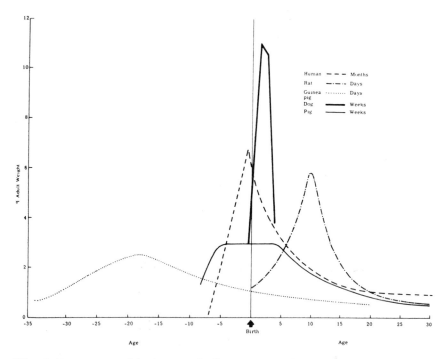

Fig. 2. Rate curves of brain growth (increments in fresh weight) in relation to birth in different species. The time scale has been arbitrarily adjusted proportionally to the average life span of each species. (Reproduced from Dobbing, J.[14])

Figure 3 shows the normal rate of brain growth in the rat in more detail. The maximum rate of DNA synthesis immediately precedes the period of maximum brain weight gain and these both occur during the second week of postnatal life.[14] Estimation of brain cholesterol has been used to indicate myelinization and it is clear that the bulk of myelinization occurs somewhat later, extending 9 to 10 days beyond the time of weaning at 21 days. Figure 4 indicates the total accumulation of DNA in various organs of the normal rat rather than the rate of DNA synthesis. More than 50 percent of DNA synthesis in the rate brain is accomplished after birth, but is relatively complete by the fourteenth to the nineteenth day. This is not true of most of the other organs of the body, which continue to grow in cell number for some period of time after that. Most of the neurons are formed in the prenatal period whereas the

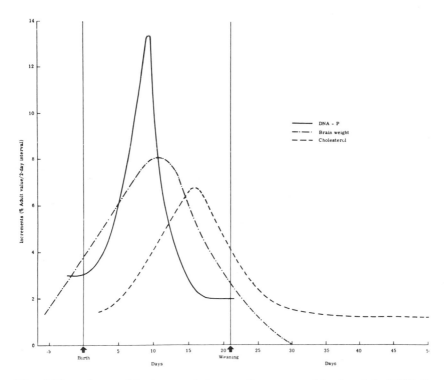

Fig. 3. Normal rate of brain growth in rats. Increments of fresh weight, DNA-P, and cholesterol are expressed as percentages of the adult value. (Reproduced from Dobbing, J.[14])

majority of the glial cells are formed soon after birth. It should be remembered, however, that some glial cells are present at birth and some neurons are formed postnatally.

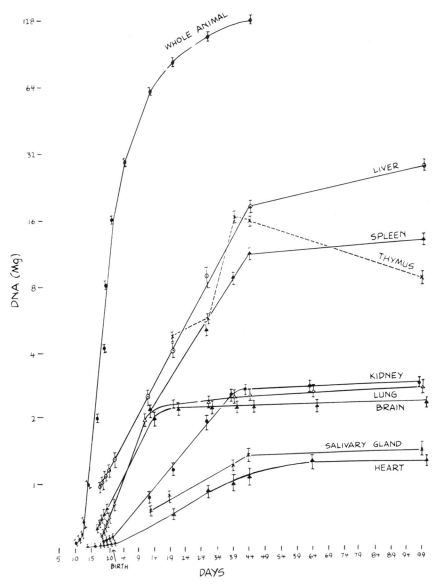

Fig. 4. DNA (mg) during normal growth in the rat. Points represent mean values for at least ten animals or organs. I represents range. (Reproduced from Winick, M. and A. Noble[15])

The Effect of Malnutrition on the Adult Rat Brain

The adult rat brain is remarkable in its resistance to malnutrition. Table I illustrates this fact. In rats whose body weights were almost halved by a 5-week diet of sucrose and water there is no change in brain weight or any measurable chemical constituent of the brain. This is a fact that is certainly not true of most of the other organs of the body. It might appear, then, that the brain is resistant to measurable changes as a result of malnutrition.

The Effect of Protein Malnutrition During the
Early Postnatal Period on the Rat Brain

What if malnutrition is instituted during the period of rapid cell growth? It has already been established that the period of brain cell proliferation in the rat is near the time of birth.

Numerous investigators have shown that a restriction in food intake of newborn rats during the period between birth and weaning (21 days) affects not only the growth rate during that period but subsequent growth when unlimited food is made available immediately after weaning.[14, 16, 17, 18, 19] There is also some evidence that severe dietary restriction in the period immediately following weaning may also be effective in limiting later growth, but it is clear that preweaning restriction is more effective.

	Control	Undernourished	Deficit
Body weight (g)	289	160	45%
Brain weight (g)	1.710	1.671	Nil
Brain composition (mmoles/kg)			
Cholesterol	49.7	49.7	Nil
Total phospholipid	65.1	66.0	Nil
Ethanolamine phospholipid	27.2	26.4	Nil
Choline phospholipid	22.5	22.9	Nil
Sphingomyelin phospholipid	5.4	4.3	Nil
Serine + inositol phospholipid	10.4	12.3	Nil
DNA-P	4.01	4.24	Nil
Whole brain DNA-P (umoles)	6.82	7.04	Nil

Table 1. Effect of 5 weeks of severe undernutrition in adult male rats on mean body weight, brain weight, brain lipid, and DNA content; 6 male rats in each group. (Reproduced from Dobbing, J.[14])

The work of Guthrie and Brown illustrates this effect.[18] A control group of eight pups per litter was nursed by a mother fed a diet of approximately 18 percent protein; the pups weaned to this same diet. As adult animals these pups reached final weight of about 480 grams. A second group of pups was raised under identical conditions except that sixteen pups were nursed by each mother. In this case the adult weights attained by these pups was in the vicinity of 350 grams. Three additional groups of pups nursed at sixteen per mother were weaned to a diet of 3 percent protein for periods of 5, 7, and 9 weeks and then rehabilitated on 18 percent protein until 19 weeks of age. The results of these experiments are given in Figure 5. It is evident that this further malnutrition in the form of an isocaloric protein deficit was also effective in limiting adult weight. Most important to these findings was the additional finding that brain weights, brain DNA, RNA, and cholesterol were also permanently reduced. These results are reproduced in Tables 2 and 3.

			Group			
	Control	D-3	D-5	D-7	D-9	F ratio
Brain wt, g	1.95 ± 0.09 [1]	1.70 ± 0.10	1.72 ± 0.09	1.68 ± 0.06	1.60 ± 0.12	21.14 [2]
Brain wt, % of body wt	0.41 ± 0.03	0.48 ± 0.03	0.51 ± 0.03	0.55 ± 0.06	0.65 ± 0.10	31.26 [3]

[1] Mean $\pm$ SD.
[2] Control > D-3, D-5, D-7, or D-9 $P < 0.01$
        D-3, D-5 > D-9 $P < 0.05$
[3] Control < D-3, D-5, D-7 or D-9 $P < 0.01$
        D-3, D-5, D-7 < D-9 $P < 0.01$

Table 2. Means, standard deviations and analysis of variance for brain weight and its relation to body weight at 19 weeks of age. (Reproduced from Guthrie, H. A. and M. L. Brown[17])

Groups	C	D-3	D-5	D-7	D-9	
No. of rats	11	12	12	11	9	F ratio
			mg/brain			
DNA [1]	3.34 ± 0.15 [2]	2.69 ± 0.29	2.83 ± 0.34	2.80 ± 0.27	2.79 ± 0.25	8.80 [3a]
RNA	3.06 ± 0.51	2.75 ± 0.38	2.78 ± 0.22	2.79 ± 0.23	2.57 ± 0.27	2.38
Cholesterol	36.9 ± 3.8	34.1 ± 3.5	29.6 ± 4.9	29.8 ± 6.4	29.0 ± 3.4	6.23 [3b]
Phospholipid phosphorus	3.49 ± 0.55	3.31 ± 0.74	3.59 ± 0.45	3.79 ± 0.79	3.17 ± 0.58	1.46
			mg/g brain			
DNA	1.72 ± 0.09	1.56 ± 0.15	1.68 ± 0.14	1.61 ± 0.15	1.77 ± 0.17	3.18
RNA	1.56 ± 0.23	1.61 ± 0.18	1.63 ± 0.09	1.64 ± 0.15	1.62 ± 0.11	0.38
Cholesterol	18.8 ± 1.7	20.0 ± 1.7	17.3 ± 2.9	17.4 ± 4.0	18.2 ± 2.6	1.96
Phospholipid phosphorus	1.78 ± 0.28	1.94 ± 0.42	2.09 ± 0.24	2.21 ± 0.44	1.96 ± 0.25	2.48

[1] n = 11, 11, 11, 10, 8 because of technical error in one day's sample.
[2] Mean $\pm$ SD.
[3] Significance of differences among group means based on Duncan's multiple range test (16).
  a. Total DNA. C > D-3, D-5, D-7 or D-9 $P < 0.01$
  b. Total cholesterol. C > D-5, D-7, D-9 $P < 0.01$
       D-3 > D-5, D-7, D-9 $P < 0.05$

Table 3. Mean values, standard deviations and analysis of variance for DNA, RNA, phospholipid phosphorus and cholesterol content and concentration of brains. (Reproduced from Guthrie, N. A. and M. L. Brown[18])

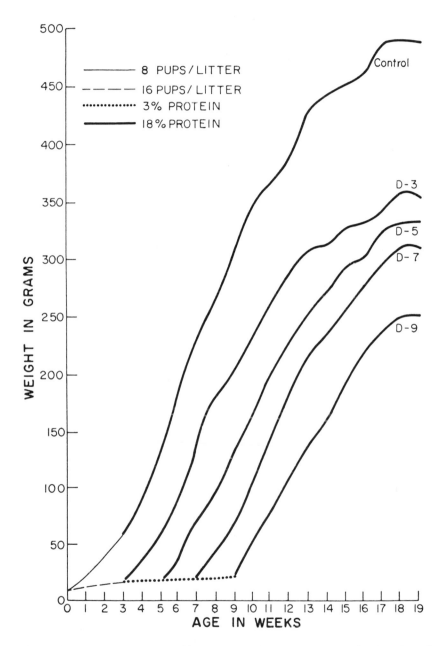

Fig. 5. Growth curves of rats subjected to nutritional deprivation for 3, 5, 7 or 9 weeks following birth before rehabilitation, compared with rats adequately nourished from birth. (Reproduced from Guthrie, H. A. and M. L. Brown[18])

Similar results were reported earlier by Winick and Nobel and more recently by Culley and Lineberger.[16, 19] Winick et al. have extended this work to demonstrate that if rehabilitation is begun at/or prior to 9 days of age (i.e., prior to the time of completion of brain DNA synthesis) the effect is almost completely reversible.[20]

Recently Barnes et al. have demonstrated that similar growth deficiencies can be induced by placing the nursing mother on a low protein diet (12 percent casein) at the time of birth with a litter size of eight pups per litter.[21]

The Effect of Protein Malnutrition During the Prenatal Period on the Rat Brain

Thus far the effects of postnatal malnutrition have been considered. Changes in brain DNA content induced during this period most probably reflect primarily changes in the population of glial cells. What can be said of the effect of malnutrition induced during the period of maximal neuronal proliferation, i.e., the prenatal or in-utero period?

Considerably less attention has been paid to this problem. Zamenhof et al.[22] have reported a decrease in body weight, brain weight, brain DNA and brain protein in the newborn of female rats maintained on an 8 percent diet (30 days before mating and during gestation) when compared with newborn of females maintained on a 27 percent protein diet for the same period of time. We have recently confirmed these finding (Table 4). Since previous to birth

	Number of animals		Offspring weights (g)		Brain content of offspring *	
Diet	Mothers	Off-spring	Body	Brain	DNA (g)	Protein (mg)
A	5	13	4.9 ± .42 **	.163 ± .019	520 ± 35	9.0 ± 1.7
B	3	12	6.1 ± .23	.177 ± .002	575 ± 28	9.7 ± 1.6
C	3	11	6.3 ± .42	.185 ± .019	560 ± 59	9.4 ± 1.6
			Decrease *** (%)			
			19%	8%	10%	7%
			Probability			
			P < .001	P < .05	P < .001	not significant

* Cerebral hemispheres, without cerebellum and olfactory lobes.
** ± Standard deviation.
*** Difference between A and B.

Table 4. The effect of restriction of maternal dietary protein on brain DNA and protein of newborns. Diet A, 8% protein ad-lib; Diet B, 27% protein-pair fed to group A; Diet C, 27% protein ad-lib. Diets were fed 30 days before mating and throughout the gestation period. All other experimental details are the same as those of Zamenhof, et al.[22]

the majority of cells in the rat brain are neurons, Zamenhof speculates that this finding probably reflects a decrease in neuron formation. Histological analysis has not been undertaken, however, so that this question remains unsettled. Whether these changes are reversible is not known. The possibility exists that what has been induced is a delay in the maturation of a certain population of cells. In this case early postnatal rehabilitation may allow the animal to compensate. If, on the other hand, there are "critical periods of neuronal development," then the possibility exists that these deficiencies are a legacy that the offspring must live with for the rest of its life. In any event, if rehabilitation is not begun by early in the postnatal period the probability is very high that this deficit will be permanent.

It can be concluded, then, that in the rat protein malnutrition during the period of rapid brain growth can lead to permanent chemical deficiencies in the brain of adult animals if rehabilitation is not begun some time before the period of brain growth is complete.

A Brief Summary of the Effect of Early Protein
Malnutrition on Learning and Behavior in the Adult Rat

The next question that follows is: Are these changes in brain chemistry reflected in changes in learning ability and/or behavior? The recent work of Frankova and Barnes is indicative of the findings of others and will be reviewed here.[23, 24] Table 5 illustrates the experimental design employed by these workers.

The day following the birth of their pups, mother rats were switched from a diet containing 25 percent casein to one with 12 percent casein or were maintained on the same 25 percent casein diet. Litter size was uniformly adjusted to eight pups. At three

Group	Preweaning Day 1-21 (dam's diet)	Experimental treatment postweaning	
		Day 22-49	From day 50
R–LP	Protein-deficient (12% casein)	Protein-deficient (5% casein)	Normal (25% casein)
R–R	Protein-deficient (12% casein)	Normal, restricted quantity (25% casein) [1]	Normal (25% casein)
R–C	Protein-deficient (12% casein)	Normal (25% casein)	Normal (25% casein)
C–C	Normal (25% casein)	Normal (25% casein)	Normal (25% casein)

[1] Only group with restricted intake; all others fed ad libitum.

Table 5. Experimental plan for nutritional deprivations during the preweaning and postweaning periods. (Reproduced from Frankova, S. and Barnes, R. H.[24])

weeks of age, the young rats were weaned. The group maintained on the 25 percent casein throughout the experiment is designated as C-C indicating control diet during both the nursing and post-weaning periods. The pups weaned from mothers receiving the 12 percent casein diet were divided into three groups. In the first, the dietary protein was lowered to 5 percent; the group was designated R-LP. The second group was fed the control diet (25 percent casein) in limited amounts, about 1-3 grams daily, to limit body weight as it was at weaning—Group R-R. A third group was restricted during the preweaning period only and then returned to 25 percent casein—Group R-C. After 49 days of life all groups were maintained on the 25 percent casein diet.

At 75 and 85 days of age the exploratory activity of all groups was investigated. Exploratory behavior was studied in an empty cage, the bottom of which was divided into eight squares. The cage was observed from behind a one-way mirror. The intensity and quality of behavior was evaluated during 9-minute test periods. Table 6 indicates the results of these experiments.

Treatment groups [1]	No. of rats	No. of squares traversed	No. of standing-up reactions	Duration of standing-up reactions	Duration of grooming	Duration of inactivity	
				sec	sec	sec	%
			Males, day 75				
C–C	11	79.2 ± 8.7 [2]	51.0 ± 6.9	68.2 ± 10.5	44.4 ± 10.8	8.0	18 [3]
R–C	8	63.7 ± 9.2	31.1 ± 6.0	39.5 ± 9.2	59.1 ± 18.7	51.2	20
R–LP	11	66.1 ± 11.2	25.9 ± 4.1	25.5 ± 5.5	57.3 ± 16.1	67.3	80
R–R	10	42.5 ± 8.4	24.3 ± 4.5	27.4 ± 5.4	45.1 ± 9.1	59.0	70
			Males, day 85				
C–C	11	74.3 ± 5.1	50.3 ± 5.0	77.2 ± 8.9	39.0 ± 10.5	12.9	9
R–C	10	44.2 ± 7.7	25.8 ± 5.8	36.5 ± 9.0	26.4 ± 9.5	84.0	70
R–LP	11	52.0 ± 6.7	46.7 ± 3.4	27.2 ± 3.8	45.6 ± 12.9	83.5	83.3
R–R	10	38.5 ± 7.8	26.1 ± 4.1	32.1 ± 6.1	59.6 ± 22.7	84.0	81.8
			Females, day 75				
C–C	8	116.0 ± 7.5	91.6 ± 8.7	148.5 ± 13.2	24.2 ± 8.2	0	0
R–C	8	115.7 ± 11.2	79.3 ± 9.6	92.3 ± 12.3	22.4 ± 8.1	0	0
R–LP	9	102.6 ± 14.3	91.6 ± 8.7	67.3 ± 11.2	46.6 ± 16.3	27.0	22.2
R–R	7	103.2 ± 16.2	51.4 ± 8.4	49.0 ± 7.9	44.7 ± 8.5	12.8	42.8
			Females, day 85				
C–C	8	122.1 ± 8.2	77.6 ± 9.8	132.9 ± 21.8	10.7 ± 4.6	0	0
R–C	8	95.8 ± 4.2	55.9 ± 9.5	91.7 ± 16.5	23.5 ± 4.8	11.2	8.0
R–LP	7	86.6 ± 11.4	47.6 ± 6.9	78.5 ± 12.3	27.8 ± 7.6	14.1	28.6
R–R	7	86.1 ± 9.6	49.8 ± 5.3	71.7 ± 8.7	53.0 ± 8.4	17.3	28.6

[1] See footnote 1 in table 2 for dietary treatment abbreviations.
[2] Mean ± SE.
[3] Percentage of animals exhibiting inactivity.

Table 6. Exploratory activity after rehabilitation in male and female rats. (Reproduced from Frankova, S. and Barnes, R. H.[24])

At 85 days of age, all recorded activities for male rats from previously malnourished groups were significantly below the level of control animals (C-C), but did not differ significantly between themselves (R-C, R-LP, and R-R). Lower values for exploratory activity was also recorded from the females from the deprived groups; when compared to the controls, however, the effect was not as strong as that seen in the males.

Learning was studied in the same groups of rats at 95 days of age in an avoidance conditioning apparatus. A cage with a plexiglass front wall and a floor of electric grids was employed in these studies. A wire mesh screen was suspended adjacent to and parallel to one wall. Again the observer was hidden by means of a one-way mirror.

The rats learned to jump onto the screen to avoid electric shocks administered through the floor grids on cue from a buzzer (the conditioned stimulus—the CS). After the CS was applied for 10 seconds the unconditioned stimulus (UCS), electric shocks from the grids, joined the conditioned stimulus and both CS and UCS were applied until the rat jumped on the screen, or for a maximum of time of 150 seconds.

The time from the onset of the CS until the rat jumped on the screen was recorded as the "latent period." Except for the first test, only slight differences were recorded between the control group, C-C, and the other groups. Most rats learned promptly to escape from the electric grid within the 10-second time interval of the CS so that most latencies were less than 10 seconds from the second test onwards. There appeared, therefore, to be no significant impairment of the learning ability of the nutritionally deprived rats.

In the course of conditioning, however, striking changes in spontaneous behavior developed in the rats that had been nutritionally deprived both before and after weaning (groups R-R and R-LP). The disturbances were manifested by changed spontaneous behavior from the third or fifth trial onward. Rats of the R-R and R-LP groups were seen to jump on the screen during the intertrial period with increasing frequency as the tests progressed. Similar results were not observed in the control group (C-C) or the group that was protein deprived only during the preweaning period (Group R-C). From the fourth through sixth test marked signs of anxiety were observed in the R-R and R-LP groups. These included rapid respiration, pilo-erection, trembling, and increased defecation.

From these and other experiments it is possible to tentatively conclude the following:

1. early protein malnutrition does not appear to significantly impair learning ability in adult, nutritionally rehabilitated rats. It should be noted, however, that the types of learning tested to date are of a very primitive type, such as shock avoidance. The answer to the question as to whether early protein malnutrition truly affects learning in the rat must await more sophisticated psychological techniques.

2. early protein malnutrition does affect the behavior and emotional status in adult, nutritionally rehabilitated rats.

3. the degree of behavioral differences tends to be greater in males than in females.

4. behavioral differences are more severe in rats that undergo protein malnutrition after weaning as well as previous to weaning.

Summary

The evidence is clear that maternal protein deficiency as well as early post-weaning protein deficiency affects the development of the brain of the laboratory rat. Psychological findings seem to indicate that these changes are reflected in disturbed emotional status and behavior in these animals as adults.

REFERENCES

1. Schrimshaw, N. S. and J. E. Gordon (eds.). *Malnutrition, Learning and Behavior.* M. I. T. Press, Cambridge, Massachusetts, 1968.

2. Schaper, A. Die fruhesten differenzirungsvorgane in centralnerven system. *Arch. F. Entwicklungs d. Organ.* 5:81, 1897.

3. Altman, J. Proliferation and migration of undifferentiated precursor cells in the rate during postnatal gliogenesis. *Exper. Neurol.* 16:263, 1966.

4. Altman, J. and G. Das. Autoradiographic and histological studies of postnatal neurogenesis. *I. J. Comp. Neurol.* 128:337, 1966.

5. Diamond, M. C., D. Krech and M. R. Rosenzweig. The effects of an enriched environment on the histology of the rat cerebral cortex. *J. Comp. Neurol.* 123:111, 1964.

6. Altman, J. Autoradiographic and histological studies of postnatal neurogenesis. II. *J. Comp. Neurol.* 128:431, 1966.

7. Altman, J. and G. Das. Autoradiographic examination of the effects of enriched environment on the rate of glial multiplication in the adult rat brain. *Nature* 204:1161, 1964.

8. Daimond, M. C., F. Law, H. Rhodes, B. Lindner, M. R. Rosenzweig, D. Krech, and E. L. Bennett. Increases in cortical depth and glia numbers in rats subjected to enriched environments. *J. Comp. Neurol.* 128:117, 1966.

9. Bodian, D. Neurons, circuits and neuroglia. In: *The Neurosciences, A Study Program,* G. Quarton, T. Melnechuk, and F. O. Schmitt (eds.). New York, Rockefeller Press. pp. 22, 1966.

10. Kruger, L. and D. Maxwell. Electron microscopy of oligodendrocytes in normal rat cerebrum. *J. Anat.* 118:411, 1966.

11. Caley, D. and D. Maxwell. An electron microscopic study of the neuroglia during postnatal development of the rat cerebrum. *J. Comp. Neurol.* 133:45, 1968.

12. Hyden, H. The Neuron. In: *The Cell,* J. Brachet and A. Mirsky (eds.). London, Academic Press. pp. 215, 1960.

13. Brizzee, K. R., J. Vogt and K. Kharetchko. Postnatal changes in glial/neuron index with a comparison of methods of cell enumeration in the white rat. *Progress in Brain Research* 4:136, 1964.

14. Dobbing, J. Vulnerable periods in developing brain. In: *Applied Neurochemistry,* A. N. Davison and J. Dobbing (eds.). Oxford: Blackwell Scientific Publications, Ltd., 1966.

15. Winick, M. and A. Noble. Quantitative changes in DNA, RNA and protein during prenatal and postnatal growth in the rat. *Develop. Biol.* 12:451, 1965.

16. Winick, M. and A. Nobel. Cellular response in rats during malnutrition at various ages. *J. Nutrition,* 89:300, 1966.

17. Barnes, R. H., S. R. Cunnold, R. R. Zimmerman, H. Simmons, R. B. Macloed, and L. Krook. Influence of nutritional deprivation in early life on learning behavior of rats as measured by performance in a water maze. *J. Nutrition,* 89:399, 1966.

18. Guthrie, H. A. and M. L. Brown. Effect of severe undernutrition in early life on growth, brain size and composition in adult rats. *J. Nutrition*, 94:419, 1968.

19. Culley, W. J. and R. O. Lineberger. Effect of undernutrition on the size and composition of the rat brain. *J. Nutrition*, 96:375, 1968.

20. Winick, M., I. Fish and P. Rosso. Cellular recovery in rat tissues after a brief period of neonatal malnutrition. *J. Nutrition*, 95:623, 1968.

21. Barnes, R. H., E. K. Neely, B. A. Labadan and S. Frankova. Postnatal nutritional deprivations as determinants of adult rat behavior toward food, its consumption and utilization. *J. Nutrition*, 96:467, 1968.

22. Zamenhof, S., E. vanMarthens, and F. L. Margolis. DNA (cell number) and protein in neonatal brain alteration by maternal dietary protein restriction. *Science* 160:322, 1968.

23. Frankova, S. and R. H. Barnes. Influence of malnutrition in early life on exploratory behavior of rats. *J. Nutrition*, 96:477, 1968.

24. Frankova, S. and R. H. Barnes. Effect of malnutrition in early life on avoidance conditioning and behavior of adult arts. *J. Nutrition*, 96:485, 1968.

HORMONAL NUTRIENT REGULATION

ROBERT W. PHILLIPS, D.V.M., Ph.D.
Associate Professor
Department of Physiology and Biophysics
Colorado State University
Fort Collins, Colorado

The cells of our body must have a constant flow of oxidizable nutrients. If this flow of available energy is stopped, for even a few minutes, cells will begin to die. Nerve cells or neurons are especially dependent on this nutrient flow and die very quickly if deprived of their energy supply. We are fortunate in that we do not have to consciously provide these nutrients. Whether we have eaten or not there is a ready, and amazingly constant, nutrient supply passing out to the tissues and organs of the body via the vascular system. After a meal, nutrients are supplied from intestinal absorption, but between meals, during fasting, and during times of emergency and stress the cellular nutrient supply is controlled and modified by mechanisms within our body. We will be concerned with the role of certain hormones in regulating nutrient flow.

There are four hormones which seem to be particularly associated with this regulation. They are insulin and glucagon from the pancreatic islets, epinephrine from the adrenal medulla, and the glucocorticoids from the adrenal cortex. Each of these hormones or hormone groups performs a different function in the regulation of nutrient flow. Yet as a whole they tend to behave synergistically and to complement each other's actions.

In many ways our bodies are like a giant industrial complex which can convert a variety of raw materials into finished products or stockpile surplus commodities for future use (Figure 1). We

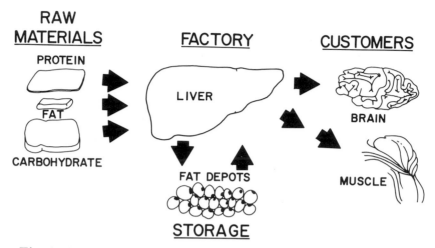

Fig. 1. Activity of the body in converting, storing and utilizing nutrients.

consume raw materials as carbohydrates, fats and proteins, which are processed in our body by what amounts to a factory, the liver, one of the most active organs in the body. Most food, as it is absorbed from the gastrointestinal tract, is shunted directly into the liver where it may be transformed for synthesis or storage, or it may be oxidized.

The liver is very active in the processes of carbohydrate, lipid, and protein formation and degradation. It is the control tower which routes nutrients out to the peripheral portions of the body for utilization. Depending on the type and amount of substrate provided via the portal vein, it may serve as the primary site of gluconeogenesis, and of amino acid utilization. In addition, it is capable of lipid synthesis and degradation. Although the liver may function very effectively as a factory and as the control site of nutrient supply, it does not in itself contain this controlling function. This is mediated by the hormones which we will discuss. They are the agents that affect change in the factory's output.

Before considering how the hormones work in directing nutrient flow, I would like to briefly review some major metabolic pathways, particularly those concerned with carbohydrate metabolism, since carbodhydrates form a large part of our daily diet. Most dietary carbohydrates enter the portal blood stream and the liver as glucose. Glucose is also the major energy source utilized by body tissues such as brain, muscle, fat depots and others. Inside cells the first step in glucose metabolism is its activation to glucose-6-phosphate (Figure 2). Glucose-6-phosphate and other phosphorylated intermediates of metabolism are not capable of crossing the cellular membrane so that once a molecule is activated in a cell, it is usually carried through

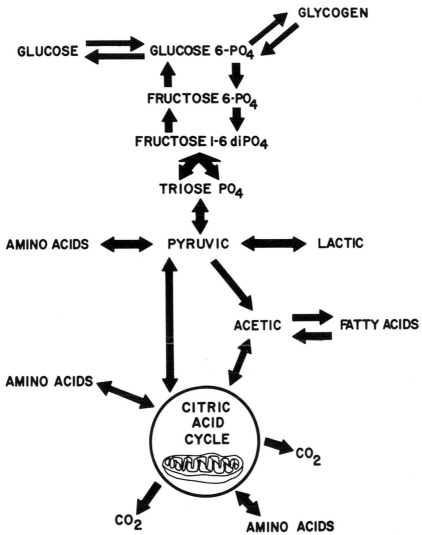

Fig. 2. Flow of nutrients into general metabolic scheme. Glucose and glycogen are initially converted to glucose-6-phosphate. Intermediates may be transformed to amino acids and fatty acids, or may be oxidized in mitochondrial citric acid cycle to CO_2. Conversely amino acids, but not fatty acids may contribute to net glucose synthesis.

the metabolic processes of that cell. The enzyme that catalyzes the formation of glucose-6-phosphate, glucokinase, is not reversible so that another enzyme is necessary for the release of glucose from cells. This enzyme is glucose-6-phosphatase. It is not present in skeletal muscle but is in high concentration in the liver so that the liver is a major source of free glucose while muscles are incapable of releasing glucose into the blood stream. Glucose-6-phosphate is at a control point in cellular metabolism. It can enter several different pathways, some of which are shown in outline form in Figure 3. By a series of reactions it may be converted to glycogen which is the form in which carbohydrate is stored in our bodies. Another sequence of reactions allows glycogen to be reconverted to glucose-6-phosphate.

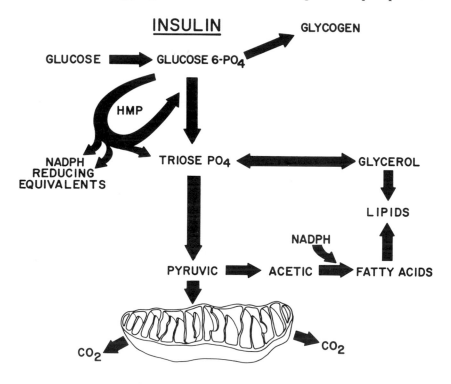

Fig. 3. Effect of insulin on carbohydrate-lipid metabolism. Insulin promotes the entrance of glucose into all metabolic pathways. There is increased synthesis of fatty acids from glucose both directly from acetic acid and indirectly due to increased activity of the hexose monophosphate shunt (HMP) which supplies the necessary NADPH reducing equivalents. Insulin facilitates glucose oxidation and increases glycogen stores if sufficient glucose is present.

Glucose-6-phosphate may enter the reaction sequence that is called glycolysis or anaerobic glycolysis. During these reactions the 6-carbon glucose molecule is converted to two 3-carbon molecules. If there is a relative deficit of oxygen, then the end product of glycolysis is lactic acid. In an individual at rest, however, most cells will not convert pyruvic acid to lactic but instead by an irreversible step will decarboxylate it to acetic acid, which may then enter the citric acid cycle by combining with oxaloacetate to form citric acid. In one turn of the cycle two carbon dioxides are released and the oxaloacetate is reformed. This cycle is found in the mitochondria and is the principal site of CO_2 production in the body. There are several other reactions which may occur; acetic acid molecules may be conjugated to form long chain fatty acids which are stored in the body's lipid depots. In addition, pyruvic may be converted to a citric acid cycle intermediate or be formed from citric acid cycle intermediates.

Many amino acids may enter our metabolic scheme, particularly if the individual is on a high protein diet or is fasting. In both of these cases there is a relative increase in the entrance of amino acids into the oxidative and gluconeogenic pathways. Gluconeogenesis is the formation of glucose from noncarbohydrate percursors. It is, in effect, a reversal of glycolysis in that pyruvic acid, lactic acid or amino acids may be converted to glucose. Several of the enzyme reactions of glycolysis are irreversible, however, so that a different enzyme or enzyme system is necessary to circumvent the irreversible step. The reactions of glycolysis and gluconeogenesis might be compared to a single railway track upon which trains run in both directions. At certain spots there is a two-rail bypass so that trains, or in this case substrates, may flow in both directions.

Of the four hormones that we will consider, insulin has been the most exhaustively studied, yet much remains unknown regarding its action on the body's cells. Its overall effect is to increase the utilization of glucose. It is an anabolic hormone. It facilitates the conversion of glucose to glucose-6-phosphate by stimulating glucokinase. If sufficient glucose is present, it also increases the deposition of glycogen in all tissues of the body and increases the flow of glucose through the reactions of glycolysis. This results in an increase in its oxidation and promotes the production of acetic acid.

There is a subsidiary pathway which glucose-6-phosphate can enter which we have not discussed. It is called by a number of names, one of which is the hexose monophosphate pathway or HMP (Figure 3). There are a number of steps in this somewhat circuitous series of reactions. The net result is the production of reducing equivalents or available hydrogen in the form of NADPH. NADPH is needed for the synthesis of fats and lipids. It transfers the H molecules to fatty acids, as they are formed. This pathway is very active in those tissues and organs where fat is synthesized, such as lipid depots, liver, and mammary gland. Insulin markedly increases glucose entry into the hexose monophosphate pathway.

Turn again to acetic acid which was formed in increasing amounts by the action of insulin. In the presence of NADPH the acetates are synthesized into fatty acids which are subsequently deposited as neutral fat after esterification with glycerol.

To recapitulate, the action of insulin facilitates glucose utilization by all known pathways and in so doing causes glycogen deposition, fat synthesis and fat deposition, and indirectly, a sparing effect on the metabolism and oxidation of amino acids and proteins. Under its action, the cells of the body increase their utilization of glucose for oxidative and for synthetic purposes.

The pancreatic islets have another hormone which is concerned with carbohydrate metabolism. It is called glucagon. It has been considered that glucagon has an anti-insulin action in the body. On a superficial examination of its dramatic initial effect on the liver this would appear to be correct. Actually we have found that glucagon and insulin are synergistic in nature and that glucagon acts to provide the increased quantities of glucose which are needed due to insulin's action. Its best known effect is on the liver where it induces glycogenolysis, that is, the breakdown of glycogen to glucose-6-PO_4 and then its release from hepatic cells as free glucose (Figure 4). This effect last less than one hour. To a lesser extent, it initially increases anaerobic glucose metabolism. Glucagon has another delayed but more prolonged action — it stimulates gluconeogenesis. Since the liver is the primary site of gluconeogenesis in the body, this effect is seen here; but it indirectly effects many tissues as an increase in hepatic gluconeogensis requires an increase of available glucogenic precursors.

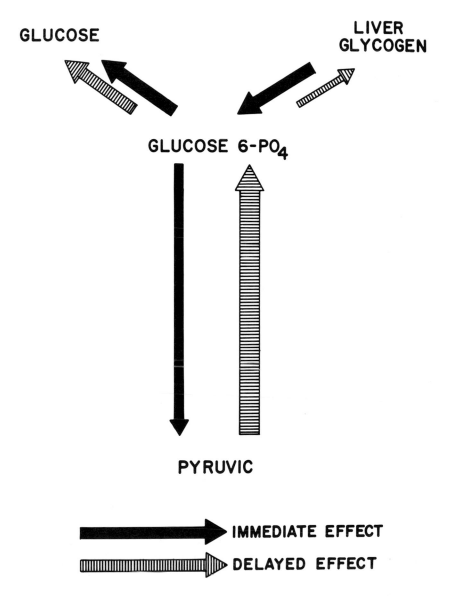

Fig. 4. Effect of glucagon on liver. There is an initial glycogenolysis which lasts less than one hour. This is followed by a more prolonged period of gluconeogenesis. Both actions result in an increased entry of glucose into the blood stream.

This delayed action acts to replenish liver glycogen and continues the increase in free glucose output by the liver, so that while insulin is increasing glucose utilization by the body as a whole, glucagon has in effect turned up the rate of hepatic glucose production by an initial glycogenolysis, and a more prolonged gluconeogenesis. This insures that those vital tissues which require glucose will have an available supply. Thus it seems evident that insulin and glucagon work in close harmony in supplying the body's cells with glucose for oxidative and synthetic purposes. As our knowledge increases we may find that these two hormones from the pancreatic islets are the major and primary controls of the minute to minute, hour by hour, shifts in nutrient supply and utilization by our body's tissues — in effect, the body's "glucostat."

There are two other classes of hormones which may greatly effect the body's nutrient utilization. Epinephrine is produced in the adrenal medulla. It can be considered as the action hormone. It is released in times of acute stress; it is the classical "fight or flight" reaction when the body metabolic machinery, particularly in skeletal muscles, is mobilized for maximal activity. In such a case muscles must have large amounts of substrate supplied to them (Figure 5). Epinephrine causes glycogenolysis to glucose-6-PO_4 in muscles which can then be utilized in anaerobic glycolysis and in the mitochondria. It initiates hepatic glycogenolysis and the release of glucose from the liver for muscle use.

Epinephrine also has a direct action on lipid depots which represent the body's large energy reserve. It increases the action of the enzyme lipase which causes a breakdown of neutral fats into free fatty acids and glycerol. These fatty acids may also be used by the muscles for energy needs and they tend to decrease the rate of glucose oxidation. One of the effects of this increased muscle metabolism particularly during vigorous physical exercise, is that the cells produce pyruvic acid more rapidly than it can be decarboxylated and utilized in the mitochondria. As a result, the excess pyruvic is converted to lactic acid and released into the blood stream. Much of the lactate goes to the liver and is resynthesized into glucose. There is some evidence that under the influnce of epinephrine there is an increase in skeletal muscle catabolism which provides additional gluconeogenic amino acids for the liver.

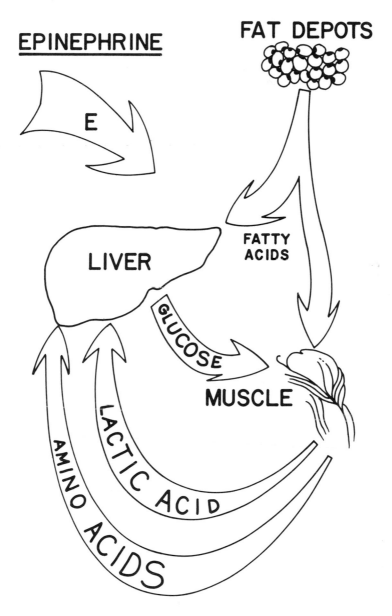

Fig. 5. Action of epinephrine in acutely supplying nutrients for emergencies. Fatty acids are released from fat depots and liver and muscle glycogen supplies are mobilized. Glucose is released by the liver but in muscle the mobilized glucose is metabolized. With increased activity, skeletal muscles release lactic acid and to a lesser extent amino acids which may be converted to glucose by the liver.

In recent years there has been an indication that under physiological conditions epinephrine may not directly initiate hepatic glycogenolysis even though it is capable of so doing in vitro. It appears that epinephrine may cause a release of glucagon which would break down liver glycogen to provide free glucose, but that epinephrine does directly break down muscle glycogen to glucose-6-PO₄.

At this time I would like to discuss in more depth one example of how hormones act to alter the supply of nutrients for cellular utilization. All three of the hormones which we have discussed so far alter glycogen metabolism. How is this accomplished? How is glycogen synthesized? How degraded? There are a number of enzymes involved in both the synthesis and degradation of glycogen. The limiting reaction in each direction is shown at the top of Figure 6. The activity of glycogen synthetase is the key to the rate of glycogen synthesis while the activity of phosphorylase controls the rate of glycogenolysis or glycogen degradation.

It is interesting that both of these enzymes exist in an active and an inactive state. In both cases the difference between the active and inactive enzyme depends on the presence or absence of a phosphate group. *The phosphorylated form of glycogen synthetase is inactive while the phosphorylated form of phosphorylase is active.* Currently it appears that glucagon and epinephrine increase the phosphorylated forms of both glycogen synthetase and phosphorylase. By so doing they tend to inactivate the glycogen synthesizing system and activate glycogen degradation resulting in an increase in glucose-6-phosphate in muscles and free glucose release from the liver.

Insulin has an opposite effect. It causes phosphate release from these two enzymes and thus enhances glycogen synthesis from glucose-6-phosphate. This is but one example of how hormones alter cellular metabolism. Not all hormone action on enzyme systems involves phosphorylation or removal of phosphate groups. In some cases they may cause activation in other ways such as by an allosteric effect or they may initiate the formation of new enzyme molecules.

The adrenal gland has another secretion which affects metabolism. It is actually a group of chemically closely related steroids; they are collectively called the glucocorticoids. Cortisol is produced in the greatest quantity with lesser amounts of corticosterone and corticone.

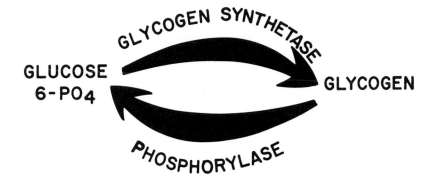

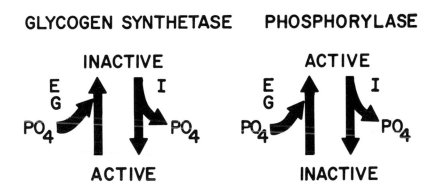

Fig. 6. Top—Limiting enzymes in glycogen synthesis and degradation both of which exist in an active and an inactive form.

Bottom—Action of the hormones insulin (I), glucagon (G), and epinephrine (E) in activating and inactivating glycogen synthesis and glycogenolysis. By phosphorylating the enzymes, epinephrine and glucagon stimulate glycogen degradation and decrease glycogen synthesis. Conversely insulin activates glycogen synthetase and inactivates phosphorylase.

These hormones have the net effect of increasing the rate of gluconeogenesis by liver cells. Actually there are a series of changes in the liver's metabolism of amino acids. Amino acid transport into the liver is facilitated. Transamination and deamination reactions increase as does the liver's production of plasma proteins and urea.

Of more concern to our discussion, gluconeogenesis from amino acids is increased, as is glycogen deposition and the release of free glucose (Figure 7). Obviously this acceleration in amino acid utilization will very rapidly deplete existing blood amino acid supplies.

The glucocorticoids also facilitate intestinal amino acid absorption and cause a degradation of muscle protein. It is not clear how the corticoids act with regard to muscle protein; they may inhibit protein synthesis as well as increase protein degradation and alter amino acid transport across the cell wall. The overall result with regard to nutrient supply for the body cells is that the glucocorticoids in times of fasting and stress increase glucose formation from amino acids and enhance plasma protein synthesis at the expense of skeletal muscle protein.

We have individually discussed some hormonal nutrient regulatory actions, that is, how the hormones affect body tissues and control cellular metabolism of carbohydrates, fats, and proteins. Of equal importance are the mechanisms which control the rate of

GLUCOCORTICOID

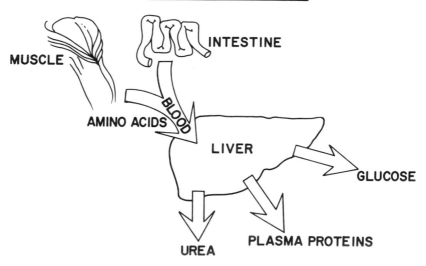

Fig. 7. Action of glucocorticoids in facilitating hepatic gluconeogenesis. Under their action there is increased intestinal amino acid absorption. In addition there is either or both decreased protein synthesis and increased proteinolysis in skeletal muscle. Amino acids are picked up by the liver and utilized for gluconeogenesis and plasma protein synthesis.

hormonal production and release. In the pancreas, insulin and glucagon are produced in tiny clusters of cells called the Islets of Langerhans. The islets contain several cell types. There are β cells which produce insulin, α cells which produce glucagon and δ cells whose function and secretion is unknown. As with most endocrine tissue the islets have a very rich vasculature. Effluent blood from the pancreas flows into the portal blood system to the liver.

Pancreatic insulin secretion is stimulated by a variety of factors, some of which are listed in Figure 8. Adrenocorticotrophic hormone (ACTH) is secreted by the anterior pituitary. Its primary role is to cause the secretion of glucocorticoids by the adrenal cortex. It also increases insulin secretion. Glucagon increases insulin secretion. This is a recent and initially surprising finding; most investigators at that time still believed that insulin and glucagon were antagonistic in nature. If we consider instead their synergistic actions, glucagon provides a steady flow of glucose for cells and insulin facilitates the cell's ability to use that glucose. On this basis it seems logical and even advantageous that glucagon would increase insulin secretion.

Insulin secretion is also stimulated by amino acids and by glucose, which has also been shown to increase insulin synthesis. Insulin release is inhibited by epinephrine. This finding seems at odds with epinephrine's glycogenolytic action. The area of knowledge concerning control or release of these two hormones is in its infancy, and I am sure that much new information will soon be available regarding both synthesis and release from pancreatic islet cells. Glucagon release is also stimulated by amino acids and ACTH. However, the main control of glucagon secretion appears to be the level of glucose in the blood stream. As plasma glucose decreases (hypoglycemia) glucagon secretion is increased, and as the blood sugar level rises (hyperglycemia) there is an inhibition of glucagon secretion.

At this point it would seem valuable to make the point that although we can inflict an infinite variety of stimuli, the glands that we are examining have a very finite response: no change, an increase in secretion, or a decrease in secretion. Because a given compound or treatment elicits a response in vitro or in an excessive dosage does not necessarily mean that it is of physiological significance in the intact individual.

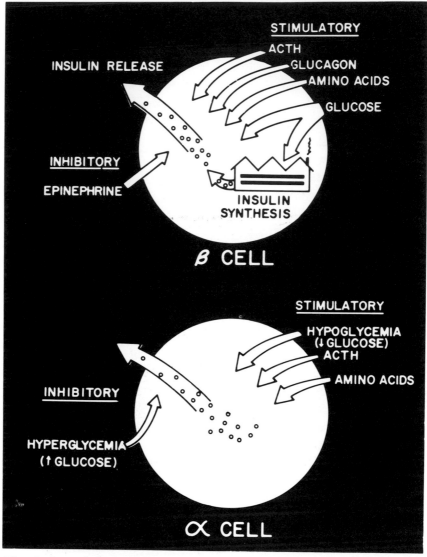

Fig. 8. Some factors which alter the rate of insulin and glucagon synthesis and release from pancreatic islets.

Adrenal medulla epinephrine release is mediated through the sympathetic nervous system. During periods of acute stress when the body cells will need extra energy, the sympathetic nervous system is stimulated and epinephrine is released. If you are to perform vigorous physical activity, you will need to consume more food;

that is exactly the action of epinephrine, to provide very rapidly more food for the body cells during vigorous activity or periods of crisis.

Glucocorticoids are released by the action of ACTH from the anterior pituitary. Their rate of release increases under conditions of body stress or fasting. Their action in nutrient regulation is of a more chronic nature than that of epinephrine.

So far we have not considered how these hormonal secretions act together to provide a constant energy source for the body's cells. Glucose is the primary substrate metabolized by the body. The glucose that is available for the cells at any given time is called the glucose pool. This pool represents the glucose that is present in the blood stream and most of the extracellular fluids. It is from this pool that glucose is continuously drawn for cellular energy requirements.

Figure 9 depicts the glucose pool and hormonal actions which modify it. Insulin acts to facilitate the removal of glucose from this pool and increases the turnover rate of the pool. Under insulin's action glucose utilization by fat, muscle, and liver cells is particularly enhanced. Increased storages of glycogen are found, lipid and protein synthesis is increased. The brain is less dependent on insulin for removal of glucose from the pool, yet its capacity to use glucose is greater under the action of insulin. Glucagon maintains the flow of glucose into the pool. It acts primarily on the liver to break down glycogen and to stimulate the gluconeogenic potential, in effect to turn on the glucose producing factory. This results in an increased flow of gluconeogenic substrates into the factory and thus, perhaps indirectly, glucagon increases the supply of amino acids and glycerol to the liver for conversion into glucose.

At the same time that fat depot glycerol is liberated, free fatty acids become available for liver and muscle oxidation. Epinephrine, under conditions of acute stress, increases the glucose pool by hepatic glycogenolysis; it also stimulates fat depot activity by mobilizing fatty acids. In the muscles glycogen is degraded, but glucose is not released. Instead, glucose-6-phosphate is metabolized and some of it subsequently released as lactic acid, which can once more be converted to glucose in the liver. The glucocorticoids supply amino acids for hepatic gluconeogenesis and stimulate key enzyme reactions promoting the formation of glucose which supplements the glucose pool.

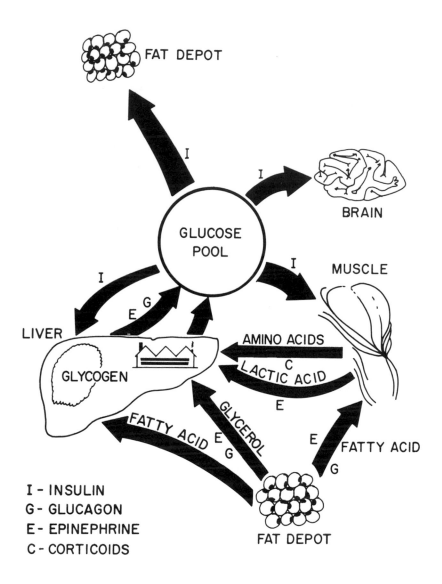

Fig. 9. Interrelationships of hormones and their actions on certain tissues in providing a constant nutrient supply to the cells of the body.

When does each act, and when does one hormone override the action of another? This is an important question and is difficult to answer at this time. All of these hormones are continuously produced and released by their respective cells. The various endocrine glands respond to internal and external environmental stimuli to alter their rates of secretion and to work in harmony, particularly through their action on the liver in providing our cells with the constant supply of oxidizable nutrients which are so essential.

SUGGESTIONS FOR FURTHER READING

Frohman, L. A. 1969. The endocrine function of the pancreas. *Annual Review of Physiology,* 31:353-382.

Lawrence, A. M. 1969. Glucagon. *Annual Review of Medicine,* 20:207-222.

Litwack, G. and D. Kritchevsky. 1964. *Actions of Hormones on Molecular Processes.* John Wiley and Sons, New York.

Marks, V. and F. C. Rose. 1965. *Hypoglycemia.* Blackwell Scientific Publications Ltd. Oxford, Great Britain.

McKerns, K. W. 1968. *Function of the Adrenal Cortex, Vol. 2.* Appleton-Century-Crofts Division of Meredith Corporation, New York.

McKerns, K. W. 1969. *Steroid Hormones and Metabolism.* Meredith, New York.

Rieser, P. 1967. *Insulin, Membrane and Metabolism.* William and Wilkins, Baltimore.

Turner, C. D. 1966. *General Endocrinology.* 4th Edition. W. B. Saunders, Philadelphia, Pa.

CONTROL OF CELLULAR ENERGY METABOLISM

DR. MELVIN M. MATHIAS
Assistant Professor
Department of Food Science and Nutrition
Colorado State University
Fort Collins, Colorado

Cells control their metabolism in order to balance their supply of nutrients and their needs for maintenance, growth, work and storage functions. The availability and composition of nutrients are a reflection of the host's dietary intake and hormonal status. The cell is capable of responding to environmental changes by sensing fluctuations of important metabolic substrates or intermediates and making appropriate alterations in its metabolism. This capability is empowered in the cell's ability to alter its diverse compliment of enzymes and their specific activities.

The mechanisms of control can be classified as: substrate availability, quantity of enzyme and allosteria. The cellular concentration of substrate along with the comparative kinetics of competing enzymes will determine the metabolic pathway taken. In other words, when substrate concentration does not saturate the active site on the enzyme, the enzyme possessing the greatest affinity will predominate. Intracellular substrate availability is controlled by membrane permeases which are, in many situations, under the control of hormones in the blood stream. The absolute quantity of enzyme protein also dictates the rate of catabolism or anabolism of particular compounds. Since the half-life of most enzyme molecules is in the order of a few days, this could be classified as a chronic type of metabolic control.

The mechanism for controlling synthesis of enzyme protein has been extensively worked out in microorganisms and is called the repressor or operon concept (Jacob and Monod 1961). The reading or utilization of genetic information (operon) that codes for the synthesis of a particular enzyme(s) is controlled by a regulator. The process is usually suppressed by the "attachment" of a repressor to the regulator. As a specific substrate increases in concentration, it prevents the specific repressor from functioning (derepression or induction) and allows the expression of the genetic information which generally codes for enzymes which catabolize the above substrate.

Acute control, which is necessary for the cell to respond to changes in environment that occur in minutes or a few hours, is afforded by allosteria. This phenomenon is depicted in Figure 1; the attachment of substrate to the active site of the native enzyme is shown in the middle. To the left is depicted the attachment of an allosteric inhibitor which has produced conformational change that decreases the affinity of the enzyme for its substrate(s) or decreases the efficiency with which it performs its designed function or both. The opposite effects happen to the allosterically stimulated enzyme shown on the right.

Not all enzymes function as control points in a particular sequence of biochemical reactions. Enzymes that do play a role in control of energy metabolism possess one or more of the following characteristics: subject to allosteric control, catalyze one-way or non-equilibrium reactions, display rate-limiting activity or important kinetic properties, require a very specific substrate or cofactors, located at a branch point between divergent pathways, or compart-

ALLOSTERIC CONTROL OF AN ENZYME

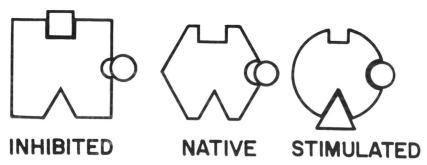

INHIBITED   NATIVE   STIMULATED

Fig. 1. Allosteric control of an enzyme.

mentalized into specialized intracellular organelles. Control points in glycolysis and in the conversion of carbohydrates to lipid and in the metabolic events that occur during the mobilization of lipid stores or after the consumption of a diet containing large amounts of lipid will be examined for examples of the above characteristics.

The glycolytic pathway is shown in Figure 2. The solid arrows represent enzymes that the cell has in excess; therefore, they perform no control function with the possible exception of the reactions that require the cofactor, nicotinamide adenine dinucleotide (NADH). Under certain circumstances the level of NADH controls the rate of these reactions. The dashed lines are examples of enzymes that catalyze one-way reactions. They partially control the rate with which glucose is oxidized for production of metabolic energy or stored as glycogen or lipid. The reverse reactions are catalyzed by separate enzymes designated as solid lines interrupted by two dots.

The enzyme that activates glucose to glucose-6-P is found in different forms that display very distinct kinetic properties. Hexokinase is always saturated with glucose, in situ. Gluckokinase has a much lower affinity for its substrate and does not become saturated; there-

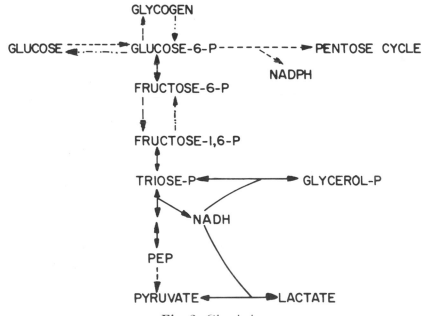

Fig. 2. Glycolysis.

fore, it it not capable of performing at maximal velocity until the level of glucose is far above normal concentrations. Thus, gluco-kinase performs an important physiological function. As blood and intracellular glucose concentration increases, the rate of glucose acti-vation increases, primarily because of the kinetic properties of gluco-kinase. In addition, the absolute amount of glucokinase activity (an example of chronic response) has been demonstrated to be dependent upon cellular carbohydrate supplies.

The conversion of phosphoenolpyruvate (PEP) to pyruvate is associated with such a tremendous loss of free energy that two enzymatic reactions are required for reversal. This will be covered more thoroughly later. The allosteric control of phosphofructokinase (PFK), which catalyzes the phosphorylation of fructose-6-P, has been extensively studied and shown to have physiological importance. It is the key allosterically controlled enzyme in the glycolytic scheme. The latter furnishes carbon-containing compounds for the citric acid cycle and for lipogenesis; these pathways are associated with sub-cellular energy production and storage, respectively. PFK is stimu-lated by physiological compounds that are low in energy, e.g., inor-ganic phosphate and adenosine 3', 5'-monophosphate, and is inhibited by compounds which signify high physiological energy, adenosine triphosphate (ATP) and citric acid.

The enzymes that are responsible for the further metabolism of pyruvate are located in mitochondria, subcellular organelles which contain the citric acid cycle and the respiratory chain of oxidative phosphorylation (see Figure 3). Pyruvate is freely permeable to the mitochondrial membrane. The key enzymes controlling the activity of the citric acid cycle are shown by the dashed lines inside the mitochondrion. They are pyruvate dehydrogenase, pyruvate car-boxylase, citrate synthetase, isocitrate dehydrogenase and alpha-ketoglutarate dehydrogenase. These enzymes display allosteric con-trol, rate-limiting activity and/or catalyze one-way reactions.

As the amount of ATP, NADH and citrate increases, and the supply of oxaloacetate and Coenzyme A (CoA) decreases, the above mentioned enzymes and the respiratory chain (indicated by NADH $\rightarrow$ ATP) are more depressed relative to PFK activity. Thus excess acetyl-CoA becomes available for fatty acid synthesis. The latter is

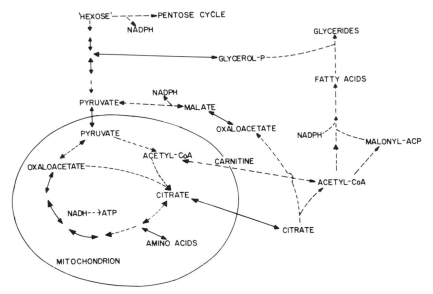

Fig. 3. Control of oxidation of carbohydrate and its conversion to lipid.

found only in the cytoplasmic compartment (cytosol). However, acetyl-CoA does not permeate the mitochondrial membrane due to its large molecular size and other physical characteristics. Translocation is accomplished via transferring the thioester bond to carnitine or conversion to citrate; both compounds are freely permeable to the membrane. Resynthesis is afforded, respectively, by transesterification or the citrate cleavage enzyme. The latter enzymic activity (part of the so-called, "citrate shuttle," see Scheme 1) has not been demonstrated in the cytosol of all animal tissues, but when found its activity has been highly correlated with dietary and physiological changes associated with hyperlipogenesis.

Other enzymic reactions that are amenable for the metabolic control of lipogenesis are shown as dashed lines in Figure 3. Recycling of the oxaloacetate generated in the cytosol by continuation of the "citate shuttle" provides reducing equivalents for support of fatty acid synthesis in the form of NADPH at the step catalyzed by malic enzyme. The source or translocation of NADH is not well understood. It has been calculated for rat adipose tissue that the "citrate shuttle" supplies 50 percent of the NADPH and the pentose cycle provides the other 50 percent for support of fatty acid synthesis.

```
Pyruvate + NAD-----------------➤Acetyl-CoA + NADH

Pyruvate⭠---------------------➤Oxaloacetate

Acetyl-CoA + Oxaloacetate------➤Citrate (Mitochondrial)

Citrate (Mithochondrial)⭠------⤬Citrate (Cytosol)

Citrate (Cytosol)-------------➤Acetyl-CoA + Oxaloacetate

Oxaloacetate + NADH⭠----------➤Malate + NAD

Malate + NADP⭠----------------➤Pyruvate + NADPH
```

```
Pyruvate + NADP---------------➤Acetyl-CoA + NADPH
```

Scheme 1. The "citrate shuttle."

This is an example of control by cofactor availability. But it is now generally accepted that the increased ability to form NADPH during hyperlipogenesis does not *push* fatty acid synthesis but is a *response* that cells make by synthesizing more enzyme protein, which takes several hours.

The rate-limiting reaction in fatty acid synthesis and the one under very definite allosteric control is acetyl-CoA carboxylase, which catalyzes the synthesis of malonyl-CoA. This enzyme protein has an obligatory requirement for citrate. Fatty acid synthetase complex catalyzes many reactions before the final production of palmitate takes place. The intermediates are attached to acyl-carrier protein (ACP); a control function has also been proposed for this protein. The fatty acids are stored by esterification with alpha-glycerol-P to form glycerides. The availability of alpha-glycerol-P in adipose tissue is related to its supply of 'hexose' because adipocytes do not contain sufficient glycerolkinase activity to reactivate free glycerol (Figure 4). This now brings us to the end of the reactions and control steps associated with the oxidation and storage of carbohydrate.

Let us now consider the utilization of lipid directly (high fat diet) or during mobilization (starvation). An increase in the intracellular concentration of free fatty acids or their CoA thioesters has been demonstrated to allosterically inhibit: fatty acid synthetase complex, acetyl-CoA carboxylase, citrate cleavage enzyme, pyruvate dehydro-

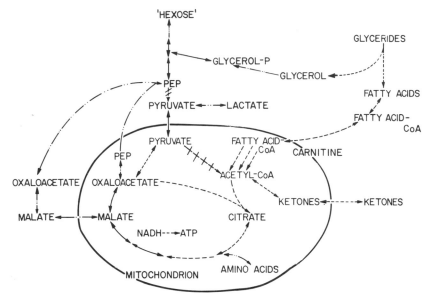

Fig. 4. Utilization of lipid and control of associated gluconeogenesis.

genase, citrate synthetase, isocitrate dehydrognase, pyruvate kinase, PFK, glucokinase and the pentose cycle. These enzymes are key points in the control of fatty acid synthesis, citric acid cycle and glycolysis. The physiological interpretation of these findings has been controversial, for the detergent properties of fatty acids cannot be wholly delineated. The control points for the utilization of lipid are shown by the dashed lines in Figure 4. Besides the above-mentioned enzymes, lipoprotein lipase, fatty acid activating enzyme, and carnitine acyl transferase may also function as control or rate-limiting steps. In liver, excess amounts of acetyl-CoA can be shunted to ketone body production — the exact subcellular mechanisms are still under considerable debate — whereas peripheral tissues possess the enzymatic steps for the utilization of ketone bodies.

To meet the body's need for 'hexose' synthesis from 3- and 4-carbon intermediates during substantial lipid oxidation, gluconeogenic activity is stimulated. The key enzymes are indicated by solid lines interrupted by two dots in Figures 2 and 4. Glycerol is only reactivated in the liver where it can be utilized for glyceride or 'hexose' synthesis. The latter pathway would be under the control of fructose-1,6-P phosphatase and glucose-6-P phosphatase (Figure 2). In order to convert pyruvate into PEP and thusly into 'hexose,' pyruvate must first be converted into oxaloacetate. This reaction is catalyzed by a solely mitochondrial enzyme, pyruvate carboxylase. Depending on the particular species, the oxaloacetate can be converted to PEP by mitochondrial PEP carboxykinase or extramitochondrial PEP carboxykinase after transfer of the oxaloacetate into the cytosol by way of malate, fumarate or aspartate (the latter two alernatives are not shown in Figure 4). These are the two enzymatic steps pointed out previously that are needed for the reversal of pyruvate kinase.

The multifunctional role of pyruvate carboxylase is depicted in Figure 5. It has a marked allosteric requirement for acetyl-CoA (indicated by the wavy line). As acetyl-CoA accumulates, it stimulates the synthesis of oxaloacetate which in turn supports the incorporation of acetyl-CoA into citrate. The latter can be oxidized via the citric acid cycle or shuttled to fatty acid synthesis in the cytosol. Furthermore, acetyl-CoA levels are well correlated with enhanced fatty acid catabolism and usually this is associated with a requirement for enhanced gluconeogenesis. As mentioned above, pyruvate carboxylase is one of the key steps in gluconeogenesis from pyruvate and its precursors, lactate and alanine.

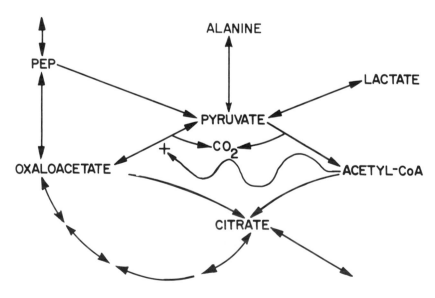

Fig. 5. Multifunctional role of pyruvate carboxylase.

It should be emphasized that all of the above processes are going on simultaneously; the relative rates of each pathway are changed slightly or to a marked degree depending upon the physiological response of the tissue. Acute adaptations that occur within seconds or minutes—particularly reactions that are subject to allosteric control—have been shown to produce oscillations in the concentration of the involved intermediates. Biochemists must utilize sophisticated computers to study models of isolated pathways and oscillations in the concentration of intermediates.

In summary, examples of enzymically catalyzed reactions that control cellular energy metabolism have been drawn from the use of carbyhydrates primarily for energy or their conversion to stored energy in the form of lipid, and then the subsequent utilization of that lipid or dietary fat for energy. Control points were shown to be subject to allosteric control, catalyze one-way or nonequilibrium reactions, display rate-limiting activity, require very specific substrates or cofactors, located at a branch point between divergent pathways or compartmentalized into organelles or particular tissues. The latter, as well as species differences, were not emphasized.

BIBLIOGRAPHY

Goodwin, T. W., ed. *The Metabolic Roles of Citrate.* Academic Press, New York. 1968.

Gran, F. C., ed. *Cellular Compartmentalization and Control of Fatty Acid Metabolism.* Academic Press, New York. 1968.

Jacob, F. and J. Monod. Genetic Regulatory Mechanisms in the Synthesis of Proteins. *J. Mol. Biol.* 3:318. 1961.

Tager, J. M., S. Papa, E Quagliariello and E. C. Slater, eds. *Regulation of Metabolic Processes in Mitochondria.* Elsevier Publishing Co., Amsterdam. 1966.

Weber, G., ed. *Advances in Enzyme Regulation.* Vols. 1-6. Pergamon Press, New York. 1963-68.

DISCUSSION

QUESTIONS TO DR. MATHIAS AND DR. PHILLIPS

QUESTION: All of the pathways for gluconeogenesis that take place in the liver are to produce glucose for use by the red blood cells and by the brain. Therefore glucose is synthesized and there is a net output of gluconeogenetic glucose from the liver, from fatty acids. This is, of course, contrary to biochemical teaching that there is no net conversion of fatty acid to glucose. Can you comment on that?

ANSWER: (Phillips) The way I interpret this is that when somebody says that you can't produce a net synthesis of glucose carbons from fatty acid carbons, it is from a sub-cellular or biochemical point of view. It is a fact that all fatty acids are going to acetate; acetate comes from fatty acids. In order to produce glucose, our real important intermediate is oxaloacetate. That is the key that will finally circumvent the PEP reaction to get us back to glucose.

So, if we are going to support gluconeogenesis, if we are going to synthesize glucose from non-glucose carbon, we are going to have to increase the concentration of oxaloacetate. We can't produce glucose if we don't synthesize excess quantities of oxaloacetate. There is only one reaction with oxaloacetate and acetate, and that is to produce citrate. All well and good, we now produce citrate, but there is one problem: the only way to go from citrate to oxaloacetate is by the TCA cycle in mammalian tissue, and in doing this we have to give off two CO_2's. So we combine oxaloacetate with acetate and we have removed one oxaloacetate from our pool that we had in the first place. As soon as we burn one acetate, we only regenerate the oxaloacetate that we started with in the first place. That is the reason I think they are trying to say there is no net synthesis of glucose from acetate.

I have one more remark. I think one of the reasons they talk about fatty acids going to glucose is that these two carbons here (acetate) are not the two carbons that are given off in one turn of the cycle. The oxaloacetate that is re-formed at this point (in the TCA cycle) contains different carbons than the ones that started as acetate. So you can get the carbons from acetate associated or found in the group of glucose molecules, but it isn't due to a net synthesis. It is just due to the cycling of the compound.

QUESTION: If you don't get any glucose from that pathway, how are you going to feed the brain?

ANSWER: You don't feed the brain fatty acids.

QUESTION: You feed it glucose, and you are not getting glucose from there.

ANSWER: That is right. The only glucose that would come from fatty acids, disregarding gamma oxidation with unsaturated fatty acids, would be from the glycerol, unless we have odd numbered fatty acid chains. Certainly those long chain fatty acids that are odd-numbered, 3-5-7, will end up with a propionate at the end. That last molecule will be glucogenic.

QUESTION: Are the three carbon sources that you are talking about now sufficient in a starved state to support the brain?

ANSWER: No, they are not. That is the reason you have such a large nitrogen deficit. There is a great deal of breakdown of body protein, and it is the glucogenic amino acids that are removed or formed as a result of the breakdown of protein that contributes to the glucogenesis that provide the brain with its food, not the fatty acids—that is, for the most part.

QUESTION: Can you comment on whether or not there is a specific carbohydrate requirement or whether we can get all the energy we need from fat?

ANSWER: (Phillips) I would say yes, there is very much a specific carbohydrate requirement. The body uses carbohydrate at a definite rate, and I don't know of any condition in which you do not get oxidation of carbohydrate, taking the animal as a whole. Certainly the degree to which carbohydrate is metabolized or oxidized compared to other substances is dependent upon the concentration of carbohydrates present or available to the tissues, because many tissues such as skeletal muscles, cardiac muscles, fat depots, may utilize not only carbohydrate but other sources for their energy need. The brain, for instance, has a specific requirement of glucose. If glucose is not available to the brain, then we go into what we think of as insulin shock, an overdose of insulin which is a dramatic lowering of the blood sugar level.

QUESTION: Can the body get enough carbohydrate out of the glycerol part of fat to meet the carbohydrate requirement when the animals are eating a high fat diet?

ANSWER: (Phillips) My thought would be no, that you would probably still be in a negative nitrogen balance in this situation because of the increased protein breakdown. I don't think glycerol would be sufficient to provide that quantity of glucose.

QUESTION: Now that you have the brain nourished, would you care to comment on how the rates of these reactions and all of the control mechanisms are involved in the storage of calories that leads to obesity and calorie requirement in the whole organism? Obesity is one of the problems that people tell us we could solve very simply if we could tell them what to eat that wouldn't cause any caloric increase. This brings us, then, to the real question of the relative efficiencies of all these enzymes and control mechanisms; can they be manipulated or are they out of control, which leads to obesity?

ANSWER: (Mathias) I think I will attack it this way. Suppose we have one person who has a real efficient TCA cycle, oxidation and phosphorylation. In other words, he doesn't have to burn much carbohydrate to supply all the ATP that he needs to make it through the day. So the rest of it is going to be stored. The question is, is there any evidence that some people are more efficient in utilizing energy, or storing energy, than others? I don't know of the experiment, but the negative experiment to this is that calories count. If you have so many calories, this is ten times more important than the efficiency with which you utilize the calories. In other words, if you have eaten 100 more calories than you need, you are going to store them. Some people may store only 90, some 80. That is unimportant compared to the dietary intake. You only get the phenomenon that you are talking about in hypothyroidism and other hormonal imbalances. There is something else wrong with this person besides the intermediary metabolism or control that I was talking about.

ANSWER: (Phillips) I would agree with Mel on that. An example is the maturity onset diabetes that we see in a fat individual. We see obese individuals who have a maturity onset of diabetes, in which there is a hyper-secretion of insulin, and I think that just the hyper-secretion of insulin in itself would lead to an obese condition if there were sufficient calories present. If there aren't enough calories, you are not going to get fat, no matter what. But if there are a sufficient number of calories, there would be any one of a number of things that might affect the degree of obesity.

QUESTION: Would you feel that there are a certain number of grams of carbohydrates necessary to provide glucose for brain function, like 40 grams of carbohydrate? There are some dietitians who prescribe a diet of 40 grams of carbohydrate, and this would be the equivalent of something like four cups of orange juice.

ANSWER: (Phillips) I am sure that there is a specific requirement or specific percentage of carbohydrate utilization that might be necessary for proper brain function, but it is awfully difficult to separate this function out. I am working with experimental animals now instead of humans. In many of these animals, it is easy to take out a liver and do a perfused isolated liver preparation, or you can do this with a kidney or various other tissues. It is difficult, however, to get an intact functional brain out, though there have been brain perfusions done. Most of them have been involved with neuro-function, not with metabolic function as far as I am aware, and I don't know of any work along this line that has specifically related percentage of glucose oxidized of this tissue versus fat tissue. I can't really give you a good answer on that.

QUESTION: (directed to Dr. Miller) You were talking this morning about having too many calories. The individual becomes obese and it is almost impossible for this person to reduce. Do I understand this correctly? That the number of cells are increased and that when you try to reduce this person you can only reduce the size of the cell and not the number? This is why they will regain their weight?

ANSWER: (Dr. Miller) That is absolutely correct. But that represents one kind of obesity, not necessarily all kinds of obesity. I suspect this is on the increase, but that is a matter of opinion. This work was done by Jules Hirsch at Rockefeller and more recently by Nittle at Mount Sinai. There is no question that overfeeding both man and experimental animals during the period of exponential growth of adipose tissue will result in increased numbers of cells which are irreversible, and that these individuals, when older, will have, in fact, more total fat, but each cell will be of approximately normal size or larger. If you take very grossly obese people who weigh as much as 400 pounds, and reduce them for extended periods of time, putting them through extensive psychological tests, psychiatry, and this kind of thing, then release them after about three years of study in ward, within a year they are back up to normal weight. For them it is their normal weight. Each of their individual cells is acting and responding and asking for more substrate and more material; psychologically and physiologically these people are starving.

Hirsch's hypothesis is that there is a form of obesity which is the result of early over-nutrition, and this is almost impossible to deal with. Now I am not proposing any more, as people did at one time, "Well, anyone who is obese is hyper-thyroid." I am not proposing that at all. I think this is a form of obesity and usually can be easily recognized if one follows longitudinally the dietary patterns or weight patterns, etc., in these people. Invariably they were much larger as babies; they were larger at warning; they were bigger children. They may not have been obese as children but they will become obese during the time of adolescence when activity drops.

COMMENT: (Beal) In our longitudinal study at the Child Research Council we found that not a single obese adolescent had been an obese baby, and, not a single fat baby became an obese adolescent.

ANSWER: (Dr. Miller) First, how did you define obese and non-obese, and what was the status used? Did you measure cell composition? Did you measure body fat, or how was this done?

BEAL: The obesity is based on a variety of things. We have bone-muscle-fat measurements, bone-muscle-fat widths from the x-rays as well as skinfold measurements. We have weight and weight per height. We have thirty different bodily dimensions. What we are talking about is real obesity, the children who are about the 90th percentile for our series in terms of weight. And the periods when these youngsters put on weight varied all the way from the child who became fat between four and seven and then just stayed fat to the child who became fat at eight or ten. There were a pair of brothers who did exactly the same thing. Between eight and ten they went from very small thin children to definitely fat adolescents. We studied the children who became fat in adolescence. We can show you any pattern you would like, but not a single one of the fat adolescents in our series was a fat baby.

ANSWER: (Dr. Miller) At what age were these measurements of obesity made in these children?

BEAL: From birth. This is a series of children whom we started studies on in the prenatal period. The first examination on the babies was done within 24 hours after delivery at the hospital. We see the babies once a month during the first year, once every three months after that until they pass the adolescent growth spurt, then once every six months until they reach adult height, and then once a year.

MILLER: These children who were obese as babies, they did not become obese even when they became adults?

BEAL: May I qualify? The study started in 1920 (the year of the original study), and took its present form in 1930. We have followed these subjects, have taken them on at intervals. That is, each year we take on new subjects, and of the ones who are now in their thirties—and we have a number of these—none of those who were fat as babies are now fat in their thirties. So we have them this far. We disagree with the Hagerstan group and with all the retrospective studies primarily.

MILLER: There is a tremendous body of retrospective studies that have been done which tend to support the idea that obesity during the first year of life will reflect itself in adulthood. In the study of adolescents it was shown that obesity appeared in individuals, and that ultimately these people became obese. If you go back in their histories you find that they were obese as infants. This is the kind of study that was done.

BEAL: The statisticians in Denver are going through with a brand new statistical method in which we are dichotomizing some of this. I hope they have the answer tomorrow. One of the dichotomies we have done is to take the average caloric intake in the first year and see whether this has any relationship to the degree of fatness in ten years or eighteen years.

QUESTION: Do you recommend any specific dietary regime?

BEAL: These are all healthy children who are living at home and the Child Research Council does nothing in the way of therapy, advice, consultation, or anything. We simply leave them on whatever regime they are on and interfere with their lives as little as possible. They are all under the care of physicians in private practice. We get them in; we test and examine them; we even turn them upside down sometimes! But we give them no advice or consultation on the side.

QUESTION: On the carbohydrate requirement, I thought that very interesting, and you brought it up. A series of papers in the *Journal of Nutrition* from Renner's group reports they were able to raise chickens on 25 percent protein—I forget the exact quantity of protein—but the rest was fat. As soon as they removed the glycerol molecule, the chickens became ketotic. In other words, rats and other animals can survive on that quantity of fat, as far as I can remember from the literature, but get ketotic; Renner's chicks do not. They survive on protein and glycerol with no carbohydrate particles ever in the diet, and I guess they grew.

ANSWER: Yes, I saw the paper given. They grew as well as the controls, which were given as much carbohydrate as they could use.

QUESTION: (to Dr. Mathias) In view of your comments about the inhibition of enzymes caused by the ingestion of lipids, would you say that we would be kinder to our body cells if we did not shift back and forth from high and low fat meals, especially since some of the enzymes are regenerated after reaching a low end?

ANSWER: (Dr. Mathias) I don't know. I have been toying with this and trying to decide how you would design an experiment to show that the enzymic deficiency is related to deposition of protein, turnover or control rates of these enzymes. Theoretically speaking, there is a steady state amount of enzymes. They have a half life. In other words, you are going to re-synthesize that enzyme every two days. However, if you are on a particular diet, you are going to re-synthesize it every three days instead of every two. So you shouldn't have to expend as much energy to do that. Theoretically it would be more efficient, but I haven't seen the experiment.

III

NUTRITION OF THE
CELL AND ORGANISM

ASCORBIC ACID METABOLISM AT MICROBIOLOGICAL, ANIMAL AND HUMAN LEVELS

LTC EUGENE M. BAKER, Ph.D.
U. S. Army Medical Research and Nutrition Laboratory
Fitzsimons General Hospital
Denver, Colorado

Microbiological

Cultures of various strains of bacteria, fungi and algae have been assayed for the presence of ascorbic acid by preparative thin layer chromatography. Within the liimts of the procedure employed there is no evidence for the presence of ascorbic acid in any of the strains examined.

Animal

"Guinea pigs, partially depleted of ascorbic acid (ASH_2), were injected daily for 2 weeks with L-ascorbic-1-^{14}C-4-^{3}H acid. The urinary excretion of both ^{14}C and ^{3}H was followed. The injected ascorbate had a $^{14}C/^3H$ ratio of 0.6. Urine activity fell from an initial value of 0.32 to a terminal plateau of 0.16-0.20, primarily due to labeled water in the urine. Metabolites of the ascorbate were isolated by basic lead precipitation, followed by chromatographic and electrophoretic separations. Numerous previously unobserved labeled components were found. Several of the urinary metabolites contained ^{3}H label only. Four or five major doubly-labeled compounds were present which were not ASH_2 but retained the original $^{14}C/^3H$ ratio. Two of these metabolites could have been uronides. The numerous doubly-labeled metabolites indicate clearly the complex nature of ascorbate metabolism in the guinea pig."[1]

"Guinea pigs were injected with ascorbic-1-^{14}C-4-^{3}H acid for one week and sacrificed. Selected tissues were homogenized and separated by centrifugation into membrane and nuclei, mitochondria, microsomes, and supernate fractions, which were assayed for ^{14}C and ^{3}H. Most activity was found in the adrenals, brain and gonads. Ca. 85% of the radioactivity was in the supernates. ^{14}C/^{3}H ratios in tissue and homogenate fractions were generally comparable to or higher than the injected ascorbate ratio, even though ^{3}H$_2$O was also demonstrated. It appears that in most tissue there is selective retention of a C-1 bearing fragment from ascorbate. Radioactivity of lyophilized brain tissue was about equally extracted by water or alcohol. Supernate radioactivity was not precipitated with TCA. Gel filtration of the supernate showed the principle labeled compound was not ascorbate and was adsorbed irreversibly on Dowex-1. Hydrolysis with β-glucuronidase produced radioactive fragments of lower molecular weight. Results suggest that labeled metabolites of ascorbate are mainly present in cell plasma as hydrophilic molecules."[2]

The above work by Karr and Scharf shows that the metabolism of ascorbic acid by the guinea pig is far more complex than is the metabolism of ascorbic acid in the human. This could explain why the ascorbic acid requirement in the guinea pig is much higher than that of the human.

Human

Most species of animals do not require ascorbic acid in their diet; but man, along with the other primates, the guinea pig, and the fruit-eating bat must have this vitamin in the diet in order to survive.[3] Man along with other ascorbic acid-dependent animals develops an illness called "scurvy" which may be fatal if the vitamin is absent from his diet for a sufficiently long period of time.

There are fragments of evidence that scurvy afflicted ancient civilizations or at least as long as records have been kept. It was described in 1550 B.C. in the Ebers papyrus[4] and writings by the ancient Greeks and Romans refer to a plague that almost certainly was scurvy.[5] Indeed historians believe that many military campaigns came to a spontaneous end because armies or navies were deprived of adequate sources of Vitamin C in their diets. Vivid accounts of scurvy appeared in the writings of the sixteenth, seventeenth and eighteenth centuries A.D. These include those of Jacques Cartier,[6] Urban Heaerne,[7] as well as Martinus Sennertus, Nitzsch and more recently Lind.[5] Many details of this devastating disease appeared in the first edition of *Encyclopaedia Britannica*.[8]

According to available reports scurvy has been rampant in the major populated areas of the world whenever the natural supplies of food were disrupted as a result of political or climatic disasters. The ancient descriptions of this disease were horrible, recalling the most obvious features, which included haemorrhagic tendencies, edema, loss of teeth, ulcerations and secondary infections.

Today, frank scurvy is uncommon, and occurs chiefly in infants weaned on to diets which are poor in ascorbic acid. In adults, scurvy may result from poverty, alcoholism or neglect, or it may occur in times of prolonged droughts and famine.

An evaluation of 33 nutrition surveys conducted by the Inter-departmental Committee on Nutrition for National Development (ICNND) U.S.A.[9] in 29 countries between 1956 and 1967, discloses that frank scurvy apparently is rare in most parts of the world. On the other hand, the intake of ascorbic acid was classed as "low" or "deficient" in a significant segment of the population of one-third of these countries and low serum levels of ascorbic acid were observed in more than 5 percent of the population of two-thirds of the countries surveyed. These same groups of individuals who had the lowest levels of ascorbic acid in their blood serum also tended to have the highest incidence of gum lesions, particularly swollen, red interdental papillae.

In view of the above, and since there has been much debate as to what would be an optimum requirement for the human, the following studies were performed.

Two separate studies of experimental human scurvy have been successfully completed. In Scurvy I, six apparently healthy men from the Iowa State Penitentiary volunteered for participation and were hospitalized on the Metabolic Ward of University Hospitals. They were fed a diet totally devoid of Vitamin C but adequate in all other essential nutrients. Two of these men escaped from the ward. The remaining four developed clinical signs of scurvy and biochemical confirmation of this. Administration of ^{14}C labeled L-ascorbic acid permitted estimations of pool size and measurement of the rate of catabolism of this vitamin. During the period of depletion there was no detectable urinary excretion of ^{14}C labeled reduced ascorbic or dehydro-ascorbic acid. The urinary excretion of ^{14}C by these subjects occurred as a first order exponential process, and in each of the four subjects did not differ from the average by more than plus or minus 2 percent despite marked differences in body weight and age. The earliest symptoms of scurvy appeared in the men after their body pools of ascorbic acid had been reduced to approximately 300 mg, by which time they were metabolizing only 7.5 mg daily. Once the body pool had been repleted to 1500 mg, urinary losses of reduced ascorbic acid begin to occur again. The rate of repletion with ascorbic acid was found to be a zero order process and directly proportional to the daily intake of ascorbic acid. Once the subjects were fed a large amount (500 mg daily) of ascorbic acid, only a limited quantity of the ingested vitamin was equilibrated with the ^{14}C labeled ascorbate pool. All of the radioactive material excreted during the depletion phase was in the form of a stable organic compound that did not behave as ascorbic acid. This organic material was separated into four unknown compounds. The observations made in Scurvy I supported the British concept that a daily intake of less than 10 mg (in this case 6.5 mg) is sufficient to alleviate and cure the clinical signs of scurvy.[10, 11, 12]

In Scurvy II a similar group of six apparently healthy volunteers from the Iowa State Penitentiary were hospitalized on the Metabolic Ward of University Hospitals. They were fed the same diet and were labeled in the same way with ^{14}C ascorbic acid. One man withdrew, whereas the remaining five completed the study.

In these men the degree of scurvy induced was more severe than it had been in the first. The clinical evidencs of scurvy included not only hemorrhagic manifestations but also edema, severe arthralgias, a peripheral neuropathy in one man and the development of the sicca syndrome in five. Repletion of the men with varying doses of L-ascorbic acid resulted in complete recovery.

In conclusion, the results of Scurvy I and II tend to indicate that an intake of 30 mg/day would be adequate to maintain normal body pool requirements of the adult human male.

REFERENCES

1. Karr, D. B., et al., *Fed. Proc.* Vol. *27*, No. 2, 256, 1968.

2. Scharf, W., et al., *Fed. Proc.* Vol. *27,* No. 2, 256, 1968.

3. Burns, J. J. (1959) Biosynthesis of L-ascorbic acid; basic defect in scurvy. *Amer. J. Med., 26,* 740-748.

4. Papyrus Ebers — Medical writings, 1550 B.C.

5. Hippocrates, Prorrhetic. lib. 2, p. 111, ca 400 B.C. Pliny, Compages in genubers solverentur ca 63 A.D. (Quoted in Lind's Treatise on Scurvy — a bicentenary volume (1953) containing a reprint of the first edition of *A Treatise of the Scurvy* by James Lind (1753). Edinburgh University Press, 1953. R. & R. Clark, Ltd., Edinburgh.)

6. Cartier, Jacques (1542) La Grosse Maladie. *19th International Congress of Physiology.* The Reynolds Printing Co. Ltd., Montreal, 1953.

7. Hearne, Urban. The First Swedish Chemist. Aberg, Bertile, *J. Chem. Educ. 27,* 334, 1950.

8. *Encyclopaedia Britannica* (1771) First Edition, Vol. 3, pp. 106-110.

9. Interdepartmental Committee on Nutrition for National Defense, U.S.A. Reports of Nutrition Surveys.

10. Bartley, W., Krebs, H. A. and O'Brien, J. R P.: Vitamin C requirement of Human Adults. A Report by the Vitamin C Subcommittee of the Accessory Food Factors Committee, Medical Research Council Special Report Series, No. 280, London, Her Majesty's Stationery Office, 1953.

11. Hodges, R. E., Baker, E. M., Hood, J., Sauberlich, H. E. and March, S. C.: Experimental Scurvy in Man. *Am. J. Clin. Nutr.* 22:535, 1969.

12. Baker, E. M., Hodges, R. E., Hood, J., Sauberlich, H. E. and March, S. C.: Metabolism of Ascorbic-1^{14}C Acid in Experimental Human Scurvy. *Am. J. Clin. Nutr.* 22:549, 1969.

THE EFFECT OF DIET ON JEJUNAL ENZYMES

ROBERT H. HERMAN, Col., MC
Chief, Metabolic Division
U. S. Army Medical Research and Nutrition Laboratory
Fitzsimons General Hospital
Denver, Colorado

Carbohydrate is a major component of our daily diet. Important sources of dietary carbohydrate are milk, bread, potatoes and flour, and table sugar. Milk provides lactose or milk sugar. Bread, potatoes and flour provide starch which is digested to provide maltose. Table sugar is chemically pure sucrose.

Figure 1 shows the common dietary disaccharides, lactose, maltose and sucrose. In the small intestine these disaccharides are hydrolyzed to form glucose and galactose, glucose only, and glucose and fructose, respectively. The hydrolysis of each disaccharide is mediated by its specific enzyme, or disaccharidase, lactase, maltase and sucrase.

Figure 2 illustrates the hydrolysis of lactose by the disaccharidase lactase into glucose and galactose. The lactase is situated in the jejunal epithelial cell surface in specialized hair-like processes called collectively, the brush border. As the lactose comes in contact with the brush border the lactase present therein hydrolyzes the lactose into glucose and galactose which are then adsorbed through the jejunal epithelial cell into the body. This is shown on the left side of the figure.

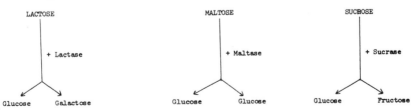

Fig. 1. Common dietary disaccharides and their constituent monosaccharides.

This work was done in collaboration with Maj. N. S. Rosensweig, Capt. F. B. Stifel, Mrs. Y. F. Herman, and Capt. D. Zakim.

On the right side is shown the situation in lactase deficiency. The deficient lactase is indicated by an X on the lactase. Lactose is not hydrolyzed because of the deficiency of the lactase. Lactose, as such, is very poorly absorbed and thus moves through the intestinal lumen pulling water from the intestine via the mechanism of osmosis. The bacteria in the colon metabolize the lactose to lactic acid. As a consequence of the water and lactic acid a watery diarrhea with a low pH results.

A similar set of events occurs in maltase and sucrase deficiency states. In man, lactase deficiency is quite common whereas maltase and sucrase deficiencies are rather rare. In some individuals lactase deficiency is present from birth and can be treated by eliminating lactose from the diet which primarily means eliminating milk from the diet. In other individuals lactase deficiency occurs as the individual becomes older. In various ethnic groups of man there is a high frequency of lactase deficiency even in younger individuals.

In the case of lactase deficiency an argument arises as to which comes first: cessation of milk-drinking and then lactase deficiency, or, lactase deficiency and then cessation of milk-drinking. To rephrase the question, does the discontinuation of dietary lactose lead to the decrease in jejunal lactase? If this were so then one could regulate the level of jejunal lactase by the administration of dietary lactose. In order to study this question it is necessary to be able

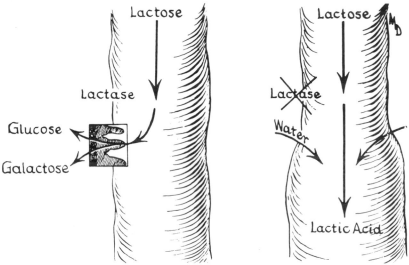

Fig. 2. The hydrolysis of lactose by jejunal lactase.

to give normal volunteers a controlled diet for a period of time and be able to obtain jejunal tissue for enzyme analysis.

On the metabolic ward of the Metabolic Division of the U. S. Army Medical Research and Nutrition Laboratory we have available young healthy men who have volunteered for medical research as part of the conscientious objector program in order to fulfill their selective service obligation. We also have a research dietitian with a staff of cooks and a diet kitchen where all types of controlled diets can be prepared. Finally, it is possible, quite simply, to obtain jejunal tissue from man by means of a gastrointestinal biopsy capsule. This is a small metal capsule connected to a long polyethylene tube which is swallowed. The capsule is moved by peristalsis to the jejunum just beyond the ligament of Treitz. Its position can be monitored by fluoroscopy.

Figure 3 shows an x-ray of the capsule positioned in the jejunum. The capsule has a small hole in it so that when negative pressure is applied to the capsule by means of a syringe attached to the end of the tubing outside of the body a small piece of jejunal mucosa is sucked into the capsule through the small hole. This triggers a sharp knife blade which slices the mucosa. The capsule is then removed quickly and the jejunal mucosa obtained. The tissue can then be frozen and stored for future enzyme assay or homogenized

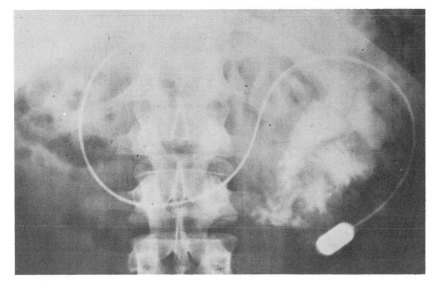

Fig. 3. X-ray of intestinal biopsy capsule positioned in the human jejunum.

and assayed fresh. The cutting of the jejunal mucosa is painless. The jejunum continually renews itself so that the biopsy site is repaired in two or three days. On a rare occasion bleeding from the site occurs to a significant degree. Out of some 1200 jejunal biopsies we have done, only two subjects had significant bleeding. If an individual does bleed, performance of jejunal biopsies is permanently discontinued.

With this brief description of the methods we can now return to the study of the problem of lactase. Table 1 outlines the protocol followed to determine whether or not dietary lactose has any influence on the activity of jejunal lactase. Seven normal male Caucasian volunteers, ages 19 to 25, were studied. None of the subjects had a history of disaccharide intolerance. A 3000 calorie liquid diet was given. The carbohydrate was entirely glucose and was compared with a diet in which the carbohydrate was entirely sucrose. In other studies, carbohydrate entirely glucose was compared with carbohydrate entirely fructose, galactose, lactose or maltose.

Figure 4 shows the results of a 60 percent glucose and sucrose diet on jejunal sucrase, maltase and lactase. In each of 4 subjects sucrase and maltase activities increased on a sucrose diet as compared to glucose. There are several jejunal maltases, one of which also has sucrase activity. It is probably this particular maltase which is affected by a sucrose diet. Note that lactase has not changed. It was found that galactose, lactose and maltose have no effect on any of the disaccharidases. Fructose however, does increase jejunal sucrase and maltase. Thus, we conclude that the active portion of

Table 1.   Protocol of studies done to determine the effect of diet on jejunal disaccharidases in man.

SUBJECTS:	Seven normal male Caucasian volunteers, ages 19 to 25. No history of disaccharide intolerance.
DIETS:	3000 calorie liquid diets. Carbohydrate entirely glucose was compared with carbohydrate entirely sucrose.

In other studies, carbohydrate entirely glucose was compared with carbohydrate entirely fructose, galactose, lactose or maltose.

the sucrose molecule is the fructose. However, it is difficult to feed fructose to man since amounts more than 35 percent of a 3000 calorie diet cause diarrhea.

Figure 5 shows the time for sucrose activity to rise after changing from a glucose diet to a sucrose diet in three subjects. Here the activity of sucrase is given as a ratio between sucrase (S) and lactase (L). This ratio gives more precise values than absolute values of sucrase alone. Since lactase does not change but remains constant, the ratio corrects for any biopsy where large amounts of submucosa are included in the biopsy specimen which has no disaccharidase activity. It can be seen that it took from 2 to 5 days for sucrase activity to increase. This is approximately the turnover time for the jejunal mucosa, i.e., the time it takes for the villus epithelial cells to be replaced by cells migrating up the villus from the jejunal crypts.

DISACCHARIDASE ACTIVITIES
GLUCOSE AND SUCROSE DIETS

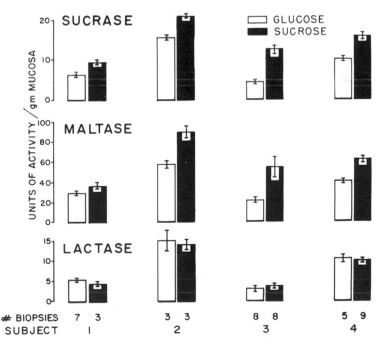

Fig. 4. The effect of glucose and sucrose diets on jejunal disaccharidases.

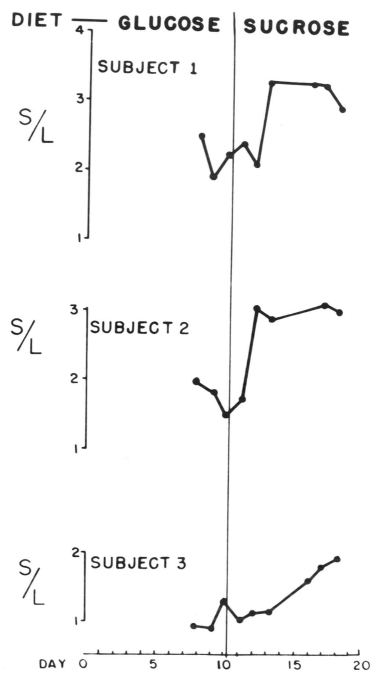

Fig. 5. The time necessary for the increase in jejunal sucrase.

Figure 6 demonstrates the fall in sucrase activity in two subjects in changing from a sucrose diet to a carbohydrate-free diet. Again, a maximum decrease in activity occurred in 5 days. From these data we have concluded that jejunal sucrase is increased by dietary sucrose and fructose and that the time it takes for this increase to become maximal is 2 to 5 days. This suggests that the presence of sucrose influences the crypt cells and the increase in the jejunal sucrase does not occur until the crypt cells have migrated up the villus to form villus epithelial cells with disaccharidase in the villus epithelial cells brush border.

Dietary lactose has no effect on jejunal lactase. From this result it seems likely that lactase deficiency occurs first followed by the cessation of milk-drinking. Maltose, galactose and glucose had little or no effect on disaccharidases.

Since diet has an important effect on some disaccharidase activity we then investigated the effect of diet on certain jejunal glycolytic enzymes. Figure 7 illustrates a portion of the glycolytic pathway and some of the enzymes that mediate the reactions. Glucokinase and hexokinase transform glucose to glucose-6-phosphate while fructokinase transforms fructose into fructose-1-phosphate (F-1-P). The F-1-P is cleaved by fructose-1-phosphate aldolase into glyceralde-hyde and dihydroxyacetone phosphate. The glucose-6-phosphate is transformed into fructose-1,6-diphosphate which is cleaved by fruc-tose-1,6-diphosphate aldolase into dihydroxyacetone phosphate and glyceraldehyde-3-phosphate. Since the specific substrate of sucrase, sucrose, increased the activity of sucrase we wondered if the specific substrates of these various glycolytic enzymes would increase the activities of these specific enzymes. That is, we wondered if glucose would affect the activity of glucokinase and hexokinase and if fruc-tose would increase the activity of fructokinase and fructose-1-phos-phate aldolase.

Figure 8 shows the effect of various diets on the activities of these various jejunal glycolytic enzymes in man. It is apparent that sucrose increases jejunal fructokinase and fructokinase activities, while a glucose diet gives lesser enzyme activities. A carbohydrate-free diet gives the least activity for these enzymes. Hexokinase and gluco-kinase activities are highest on the glucose diet. Fructose-1,6-diphos-

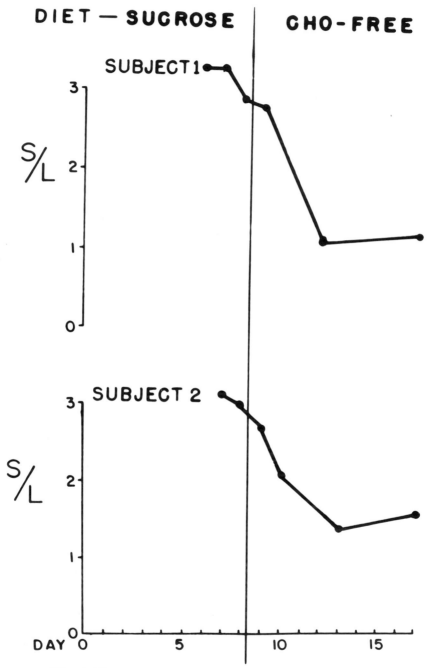

Fig. 6. The time necessary for the decrease in jejunal sucrase.

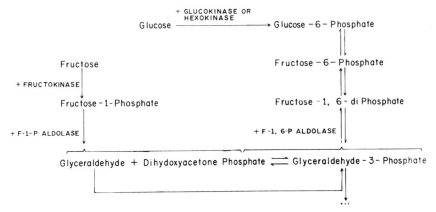

Fig. 7. A portion of the glycolytic pathway and some of the enzymes involved in some of the steps.

GLYCOLYTIC ENZYMES — HUMAN JEJUNUM

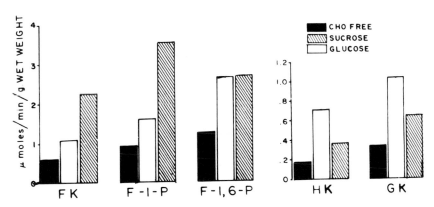

Fig. 8. The effect of diet on human jejunal glycolytic enzymes: fructokinase (FK), fructose-1-phosphate aldolase (F-1-P), fructose-1,6-diphosphate aldolase (F-1,6-P), hexokinase (HK) and glucokinase (GK).

phate aldolase activity is increased equally by dietary glucose and sucrose.

Figure 9 shows the time response of one of the glycolytic enzymes, fructokinase. In two subjects on a sucrose diet jejunal fructokinase increased in one day. In subject 3 an increase occurred in 1 day and became maximal by the third day. Upon discontinuation of

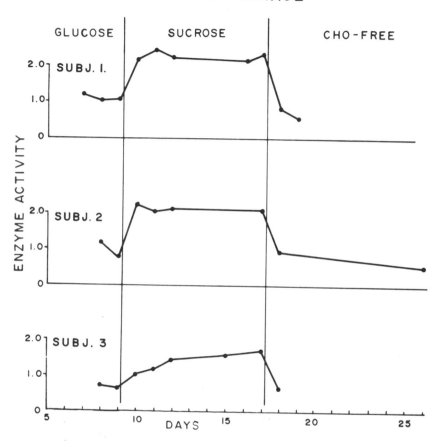

Fig. 9. The time response of jejunal fructokinase to a sucrose diet.

the sucrose diet the fructokinase activity decreased in all three subjects within one day.

From these data we can conclude the following. There appear to be at least two types of adaptive responses to diet in the human jejunum: 1) There is a direct response of the glycolytic enzymes of each epithelial cell to changes in the diet. 2) There is a delayed adaptive response of disaccharidase activity which probably acts via the crypt cell and intestinal cell turnover.

During the course of these studies we had occasion to study a patient with tropical sprue. This is a disease which typically occurs in individuals living in or visiting certain tropical and semi-tropical countries such as Puerto Rico and the countries of Southeast Asia. It results in a chronic diarrheal state, weight loss and malabsorption of dietary constituents. Microscopic examination of the intestinal mucosa obtained by biopsy reveals a very abnormal mucosa with loss of villus structure. The etiology of the disease is unknown. However, it is known that many of these patients develop a megaloblastic anemia which is specifically treatable by folic acid. It is thought that dietary folic acid is not absorbed properly because of the structural abnormalities of the intestinal mucosa.

A deficiency of folic acid, per se, is not thought to be the specific cause of the disease. Nevertheless, folic acid is the specific treatment for tropical sprue. Often, the antibiotic tetracycline is used in addition for therapy since the patients seem to do better when tetracycline and folic acid are used together. However, tetracycline alone is not adequate therapy for tropical sprue. But, because of the efficacy of tetracycline and folic acid in the therapy of tropical sprue some investigators subscribe to the idea that there are microorganisms in the intestinal tract that are in some way involved in the etiology of tropical sprue.

Because our patient with tropical sprue had an abnormal jejunal mucosa we wondered whether his jejunal glycolytic enzymes would respond to diet in the same way as our normal subjects The response of this patient's enzymes to dietary carbohydrate was very poor indeed. Because folic acid is a specific treatment for tropical sprue we then decided to test the effect of folic acid on the patient's jejunal enzymes. Oral folic acid caused a marked increase in the activities of all of the glycolytic enzymes. The increases were so pronounced that we embarked on a study of the effect of folic acid on jejunal enzymes in normal subjects and in obese patients undergoing weight reduction by fasting.

Figure 10 shows the effect of oral folic acid, 5 mg. given three times per day, to obese fasting patients. It can be seen that folic acid increased all of the jejunal glycolytic enzyme activities even during fasting and that the effect is additive with the effect of diet.

Figure 11 shows the effect of oral folic acid in normal subjects. All of the enzyme activities increased above the values seen with just

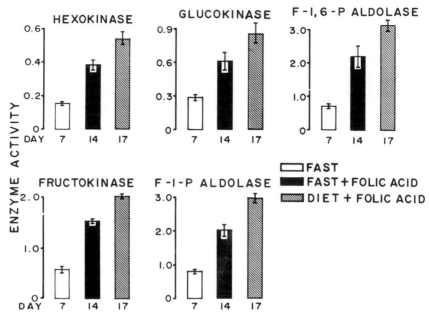

Fig. 10. The effect of folic acid on jejunal glycolytic enzymes in obese, fasting patients.

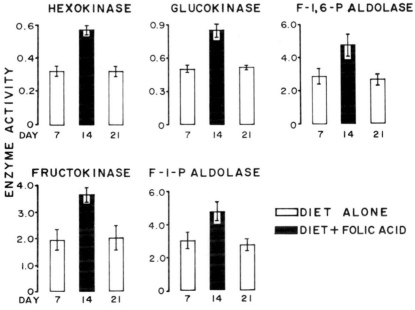

Fig. 11. The effect of folic acid on jejunal glycolytic enzymes in normal male subjects.

diet alone. We then tested the effect of oral folic acid, intramuscular folic acid and Vitamin B_{12}. Vitamin B_{12} is able to correct the megaloblastic anemia seen in pernicious anemia. Folic acid also will reverse the anemia of pernicious anemia. Thus, there seems to be some relationship between folic acid and Vitamin B_{12} though the nature of this relationship is obscure.

Figure 12 illustrates the effect of oral folic acid on jejunal glucokinase activity. The increase of glucokinase activity is well demonstrated. Intramuscular folic acid, however, caused no change whatever. Oral Vitamin B_{12} also had no effect on glucokinase activity. Similarly, intramuscular folic acid and oral Vitamin B_{12} had no effect on any other of the glycolytic enzyme activities.

We also tested the effect of oral folic acid on the jejunal disaccharidases. This is shown in Figure 13. Oral folic acid had no effect on jejunal lactase, sucrase or maltese whether the data is expressed in absolute values or as a ratio. We also compared the effect of oral folic acid on jejunal enzymes with the level of serum folic acid.

Figure 14 shows that jejunal fructokinase increases with oral folic acid and that the serum folate level increases as well. When oral folic acid was discontinued the jejunal fructokinase activity promptly decreased while the serum folate level remained elevatd. So we can say that the effect of folic acid on jejunal glycolytic enzyme activity

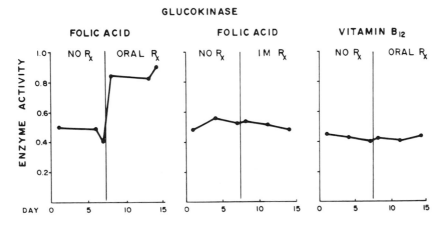

Fig. 12. Effect of oral and intramuscular folic acid and oral vitamin B_{12} on jejunal glucokinase.

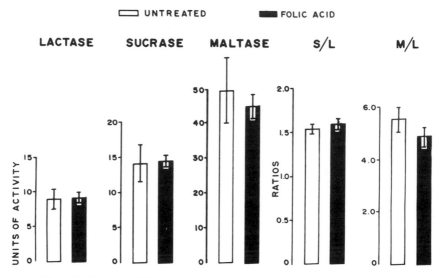

Fig. 13. Lack of effect of oral folic acid on jejunal disaccharidases.

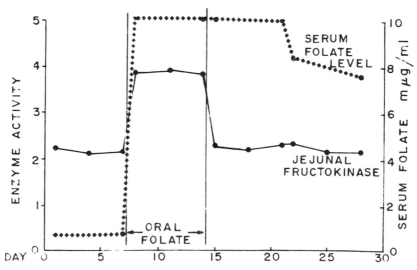

Fig. 14. The correlation of the response of jejunal fructokinase to oral folic acid with serum folate levels.

is a direct effect on the jejunal epithelial cells and does not depend on the level of serum folate.

In Figure 15 is shown the dose response of hexokinase and fructose-1,6-diphosphate aldodase to folic acid. With a dose of oral folic acid of 100 μg the enzyme activities increase. As the dose is increased there is a corresponding increase in enzyme activity.

Figure 16 shows the effect of varying doses of folic acid on fructokinase fructose-1-phosphate aldolase activities. Again with increasing doses of folic acid there is a corresponding increase in enzyme activities. A small but definite increase is seen in enzyme activities with a dose of 100 μg of folic acid per day.

Thus, in addition to the effects of dietary carbohydrate on jejunal enzymes there is an effect of oral folic acid on jejunal glycolytic enzymes. We have been able, also, to demonstrate a similar effect of dietary galactose on human jejunal galactose metabolizing enzymes.

What can we say about the mechanism of action of dietary carbohydrate and oral folic acid in increasing jejunal enzyme activity? At present, our working hypotheses are that dietary sucrose affects the jejunal crypt cells. This effect does not become manifest until the crypt cells have migrated up the jejunal villus and have devel-

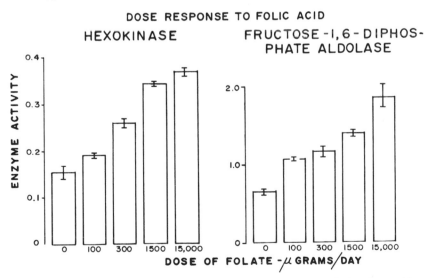

Fig. 15. The response of jejunal hexokinase and fructose-1,6-diphosphate aldolase to varying doses of oral folic acid.

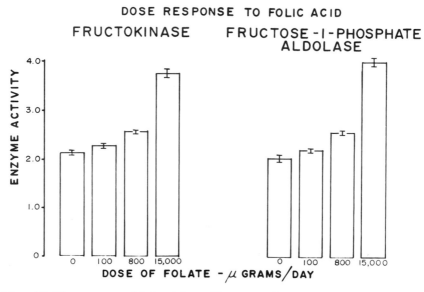

Fig. 16. The response of jejunal fructokinase and fructose-1-phosphate aldolase to varying doses of oral folic acid.

oped a brush border which is the locus of jejunal disaccharidases. Dietary glucose and fructose or sucrose affect the jejunal epithelial cells of the villus directly and in some way "induce," i.e., increase the synthesis of, the enzymes involved in the specific metabolism of these sugars. Folic acid in microorganisms, and in man, is metabolized to a cofactor form, N^{10}-formyltetrahydrofolic acid. This cofactor is necessary to form N-formylmethionyl-transfer ribonucleic acid or N-formylmethionyl tRNA. In microorganisms this N-formylmethionyl tRNA is necessary to initiate protein synthesis. We believe that this mechanism also occurs in man, at lease for some enzymes. By providing oral folic acid we postulate that increased amounts of N-formylmethionyl tRNA is generated leading to increased protein synthesis and hence increased enzyme synthesis at the ribosomal level.

These types of studies show clearly that the metabolism of the intestinal cells of man is greatly influenced by the type and amount of dietary substances. The metabolism of the intestinal epithelial cells is important in the proper functioning of the intestinal tract and this metabolism then is regulated partly by what we eat.

GENERAL REFERENCES

Rosensweig, N. S. and R. H. Herman. The control of jejunal sucrase and maltase activity in man by dietary sucrose or fructose. A model for the study of enzyme regulation in man. *J. Clin. Invest.* 47:2253, 1968.

Stifel, F. B., R. H. Herman and N. S. Rosensweig. Dietary regulation of galactose-metabolizing enzymes: Adaptive changes in rat jejunum. *Science* 162:692, 1968.

Stifel, F. B., N. S. Rosensweig, D. Zakim, and R. H. Herman. Dietary regulation of glycolytic enzymes. I. Adaptive changes in rat jejunum. *Biochim. Biophys. Acta* 170:221, 1968.

Rosensweig, N. S., F. B. Stifel, R. H. Herman and D. Zakim. Dietary regulation of glycolytic enzymes. II. Adaptive changes in human jejunum. *Biochim. Biophys. Acta* 170:228, 1968.

Rosensweig, N. S. and R. H. Herman. Time response of jejunal sucrase and maltase activity to a high sucrose diet in normal man. *Gastroenterology* 56:500, 1969.

Stifel, F. B., R. H. Herman and N. S. Rosensweig. Dietary regulation of glycolytic enzymes. III. Adaptive changes in rat jejunal pyruvate kinase, phosphofructokinase, fructose disphosphatase and glycerol-3-phosphate dehydrogenase. *Biochim. Biophys. Acta* 184:29, 1969.

Rosensweig, N. S., R. H. Herman, F. B. Stifel and Y. F. Herman. The regulation of human jejunal glycolytic enzymes by oral folic acid. *J. Clin. Invest.,* in press.

DISCUSSION

QUESTIONS TO DR. BAKER AND DR. HERMAN

QUESTION: In your work with lactase deficiencies, have you found that there are gradations or does the diet have to be completely lactose free?

ANSWER: (Dr. Herman) Certainly there are degrees of lactase deficiency. There are many people with lactase deficiency who eat a little bit of ice cream or something of this sort. Certainly it is a dose phenomena. What we clinically do, because we don't want to do a mass screening program with intestinal biopsies on everybody — it is very difficult, sometimes, technically to handle a lot of people since there is a lot of time involved — we administer lactose to people at 100 grams just as though we were doing a glucose tolerance test. But instead we substitute lactose and do a lactose tolerance test. A hundred grams will cause symptoms in many people with a mild lactase deficiency, and watery diarrhea with the people with the moderately severe form, and extremely severe diarrhea and abdominal cramping and symptoms that last several days with people who have a very severe deficiency. So, for a severe deficiency, we would give people maybe 30 or 50 grams. It is a dose phenomena, the greater the degree of deficiency, the more the symptoms. It is possible to take small amounts, yes.

QUESTION: I also would like your opinion. I have read on disaccharidase deficiencies in certain journals, that products like yogurt and buttermilk are actually lactose free. Is that correct?

ANSWER: I can't tell you about yogurt or buttermilk; I know skimmed milk has lactose in it. I don't know about yogurt. We have really not had occasion to look into that. Certain cheese products will have lactose in them. I wouldn't be able to give you exactly what the analysis shows. I would suspect that there is a variable content since I don't believe the commercial production of yogurt is that well standardized.

RESPONSE: The reason I am asking that is there are certain physicians who do order a completely lactose free diet, but then they add things like yogurt, buttermilk, and cheese because lactose is water soluble, and patients really question this. I am searching for a definite answer.

ANSWER: (Dr. Herman) I think the point is that lactose can be trapped in many of these products even though it is water soluble, and they don't take special efforts to make sure that it is washed free. So I would imagine that there are amounts in there; I would imagine that they are relatively small amounts, and since small amounts can be tolerated, it might be essentially lactose free, but not absolutely.

QUESTION: Since we are all sitting here wondering if we are about to develop a lactase deficiency, what percentage of the population might we expect to have a deficiency?

ANSWER: (Dr. Herman) Most of the people in the world are lactase deficient, most of the Orientals, many groups of Negroes. These are the groups that have been most studied. Probably people from the Pacific areas, probably the people in India are lactase deficient. There is a greater frequency in these ethnic groups; in Caucasians the frequency of deficiency is less. However, the problem with this is that it hasn't been screened this much, and I would suspect that if one studied different ethnic Caucasian populations, he might find a variable frequency of deficiency. This is sometimes difficult to do. At the present what is believed is that Orientals and Negroes probably have a higher degree of lactase deficiency and Caucasians have less frequency. But nevertheless there are plnty of Caucasians who are lactase deficient. This often will develop in Caucasians at a later age, so there is a higher frequency in middle-aged people, middle-aged Caucasians, rather than younger Caucasians. Whereas let us say in Negroes or Orientals the lactase deficiency occurs at a much younger age, and this may well account for the fact that in many Oriental cultures and Negro cultures, there is an absence of milk. This is probably very physiologic for them.

QUESTION: When you mentioned that the Oriental people have more of a lactase deficiency, I wondered about our wisdom of sending powdered milk and evaporated milk to the Orientals.

ANSWER: (Dr. Herman) That is, of course, a particular problem when you are trying to deal with malnutrition, and one of the nice sources of protein and carbohydrate is milk or dried milk product. Often this is sent to be given to children, and children are less likely to be lactase deficient. But one must be very careful when he does send such milk products to treat malnutrition that he doesn't run into difficulty because of lactase deficiency; this should be recognized.

What we should try to do is provide some form of protein and carbohydrate which is more closely akin to the usual food that is taken in by the culture. Of course, this is not possible to do, and what this really points up is that in different ethnic groups there are different food preferences, probably in many cases on a physiologic basis, and we should investigate what is the proper dietary source of food for different ethnic groups. It may not necessarily be all the same.

It is the old story—what is one man's meat is another man's poison—and people do vary. We are all of the same genetic race, but there are variations among people even within the same ethnic group. So what we are talking about are gene frequencies, and we have to study more what the ethnic variations in food tolerance are. This is a subject that has hardly been studied because most people assumed that everybody should be able to eat what everybody else eats, and this is not true.

QUESTION: (to Dr. Baker) As I understood it in the depletion studies with ascorbic acid, the loss of ascorbic acid amounted to about 2.6 percent per day.

ANSWER: (Dr. Baker) Yes, that is absolutely true. As I said in the first Iowa City Study, the figure was 2.6 percent of the body pool. The second Iowa City Study, the figure turned out to be 1.55 percent, really no statistical difference there at all, and there was less than a 1 percent overall variation comparing all nine subjects.

QUESTION: And this also continued after unlabeled ascorbic acid was added in large doses?

ANSWER: (Dr. Baker) Yes, this was a point that I wanted to make in the so-called Scurvy I, that when the unlabeled ascorbic acid was fed at the same level but without the isotope, the decay curve was the same as it had been during the deficient period.

QUESTION: In this case then, would you consider it possible that the decay or the loss of ascorbic acid was entirely independent of the body functions or needs?

ANSWER: (Dr. Baker) The loss or the decay had nothing at all to do with the function of the ascorbate in the body. It doesn't even imply function.

QUESTION: Therefore, in the function of the ascorbic acid in the body, it is probably the catalyst, in that there would be no metabolic process or products?

ANSWER: (Dr. Baker) There is no known process outside of a hypothesis of what might be a specific function of ascorbic acid. I think Dr. Herman has just given you one excellent example;

certainly insofar as hydroxylation of hydroxyproline is concerned, ascorbic acid does enhance activity within the system, but it does not do so enzymically or co-enzymically in view of the fact that the four di-sterio isomers will show equal activity.

QUESTION: Perhaps it is more of a function of its reductive power then?

ANSWER: (Dr. Baker) I'd say the function is probably closer to that of a control function. If you would, you might consider ascorbic acid, if one wants to be heretical, a water-soluble hormone.

QUESTION: (to Dr. Herman) You have been working with young adults, and since lactase seems to be going down in activity throughout life, if it was considered as an adaptive enzyme, is there adaptation by the neonate? I realize you haven't been working with the neonates, but do you know any work along this line?

ANSWER: (Dr. Herman) There has been a lot of speculation that this might be the case. As far as I know, nobody has been able to prove in man that by continual feeding of lactose, you can influence lactase at all. We have tried and have not been successful. We have fed lactose for long periods of time to men; we have also fed galactose in very large amounts, and here of course, you have to be careful because there are a number of people who have galactosemia as heterozygote. So if you give very large amounts of galactose, they suddenly come in and complain of blurred vision. Therefore, before we do any of these studies now, we measure all of the galactose enzymes in the red blood cells just to be sure we don't inadvertently give somebody too much galactose, more than he can tolerate.

But galactose itself doesn't have any effect on lactase, and if you look through the literature, this has been tried in a number of studies, and it is very difficult. Most people have not been successful in increasing it. This has not been studied in infants, of course, but the suggestion is that ordinarily we are born with a certain amount of lactase, and then when we get weaned at some variable period, the enzyme decays and can never be induced. The gene that regulates lactase production is turned off. We don't know how it is turned off or why it is kept turned off, why it can't be turned on again, but it is apparently an example of an aging process where an enzyme synthesis is turned off and can't be restarted. They have tried in certain animals to increase lactase by giving galactose or lactose and have also been unsuccessful. So apparently there is no way to turn it back on once it is turned off.

QUESTION: What if a young animal or young individual was kept on a high lactase diet from birth? In other words, would it maintain its high level of lactase activity?

ANSWER: (Dr. Herman) This has been suggested by a number of people, and I don't know that it has ever been tried in man. I think it has been tried in animals, and as far as I know, this hasn't been successful. But the number of studies where this has been done are very limited. There are some people who have pointed out that if you keep animals on lactose for a very long period of time, ultimately there will be some increase in lactase. I am not sure that everybody believes this data, so as far as I can tell at the moment, there is no evidence to show that you can do this.

MEDICINE AND THE HUMAN CHROMOSOMES

DR. ARTHUR ROBINSON
University of Colorado Medical Center
Department of Biophysics
4200 East Ninth Avenue
Denver, Colorado

A new era in cytogenetics was initiated by Tjio and Levan[1] in 1956 with the discovery that the number of human chromosomes is 46, and not 48 as was previously believed (Figures 1a and 1b). The thirteen years since then have witnessed a continuous and exponential increase in our knowledge of the human chromosomes, which has had sufficient impact both on fundamental biology and on medicine to weld the two more closely than ever before.

Techniques have been developed which make possible examination of the karyotype of cells obtained from most tissues in the body. In most cases, in vitro culture of the tissue is required in order to collect a sufficient number of mitotic figures capable of being analyzed.[2] When, however, one wishes to avoid in vitro culture, which, in the case of a mixture of cell populations (mosaicism), might permit the selective overgrowth of one population of cells at the expense of another, it is possible to examine bone marrow biopsies directly, since this tissue usually contains sufficient numbers of mitoses in vivo.[3]

One of the results of the new knowledge in this field has been the realization that man is subject to all of the chromosomal abnormalities, both numerical and structural, that have previously been found

From the Eleanor Roosevelt Institute for Cancer Research and the Florence R. Sabin Research Laboratories of the Department of Biophysics (Contribution No. 375), University of Colorado Medical Center, Denver. This investigation was aided by U. S. Public Health Service grant HD 00622 and a grant from the Genetic Foundation.

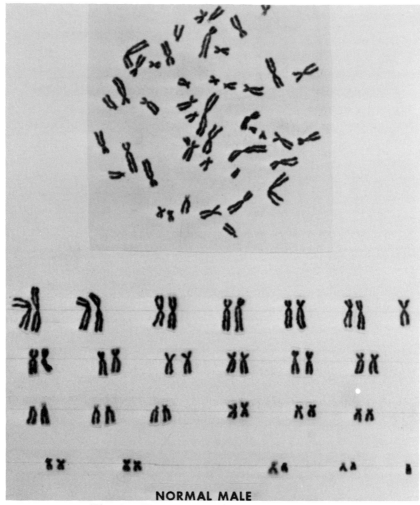

NORMAL MALE

Fig. 1a. Human chromosomes, normal male.

in other living organisms — both in plants and animals. One has the impression, thus far unverified, that these aberrations may be even more frequent in man. Indeed, the role of chromosomal abnormalities in clinical medicine is now so well recognized that most clinical centers have a laboratory devoted to their study.

The constancy of chromosomal number and structure in the human karyotype was pointed out early in the development of human cytogenetics.[4] Unexpected, however, was the high frequency of patho-

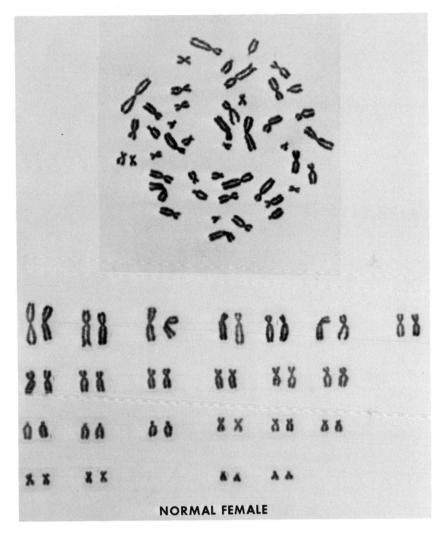

NORMAL FEMALE

Fig. 1b. Human chromosomes, normal female.

logical states that have been found to be associated with gross abnormalities of the chromosomes. It has been estimated that 10 percent of all fertilized eggs, 40 percent of spontaneous abortions, and 1 percent of newborn babies have gross malformations of their chromosomes.[5]

There are two general types of aberrations.[6] One is structural, due to chromosomal breakage, with or without abnormal reunion,

and resulting in deletions, translocations, isochromosomes, ring chromosomes and pericentric inversions being found in a variety of conditions. The role of viruses, drugs, and high energy radiation in producing chromosomal breakage is a matter of great current concern.

The other type of aberration, probably more common and more
serious in its pathological effects, is due to the presence of an extra
or missing chromosome, a phenomenon resulting from either meiotic
or mitotic nondisjunction. At least 0.5 percent of all newborn
babies may be aneuploid.

It is noteworthy that chromosomal imbalance involving the autosomes is much less readily tolerated than that involving the sex
chromosomes, so that for the occasional case where aneuploidy due
to an autosome permits a live birth, the baby has extremely serious
involvement, the mildest example of which is Down's syndrome
(Trisomy 21).

Since the discovery by Barr[7] that a dimorphism exists in cells
examined from the two sexes, it has been evident that the X chromosome has some unusual and individual properties. Twenty percent
or more of cells scraped from the buccal mucous membranes of
chromosomally normal females contain a deep staining chromatin
body in the nucleus, the Barr body, which probably represents the
late replicating and at least partially genetically inactive member of
the X chromosome pair (Figure 2).

The hypothesis (Russell-Lyon) that the female represents a mosaic
of clones of X chromosomal activity,[8a, b] by now supported by a considerable amount of evidence, has as its corollary that most cells,
male or female, will usually have only one completely genetically
active X chromosome, the rest of the X chromosomes forming chromatin bodies (Figure 3). The observation, therefore, that the number
of chromatin bodies in somatic cells is equal to one less than the
number of X chromosomes provides the basis for a simple screening
test for determining the X chromosomal constitution of any individual.
The hypothesis also provides a saitsfactory explanation for the phenomenon of dosage compensation for sex-linked genes.

The Barr test can, therefore, be readily applied to large numbers
of persons, in order to make possible a means of studying the frequency of non-disjunction of the X chromosome in human popu-

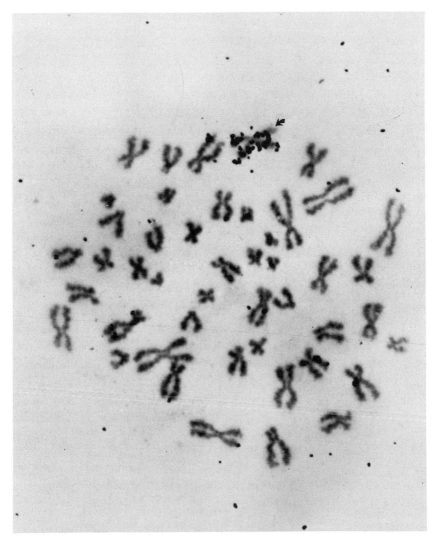

Fig. 2. Human mitosis. One chromosome (arrow) is heavily labelled with tritiated thymidine. This is assumed to be the late replicating X chromosome that forms the Barr body.

lation. To the extent that such occurrences mirror the frequency of non-disjunction among all chromosomes, this test might provide information on the epidemiology of numerical chromosomal aberrations in general in these populations, and eventually disclose some of the causes of this significant factor in fetal wastage and human disease.

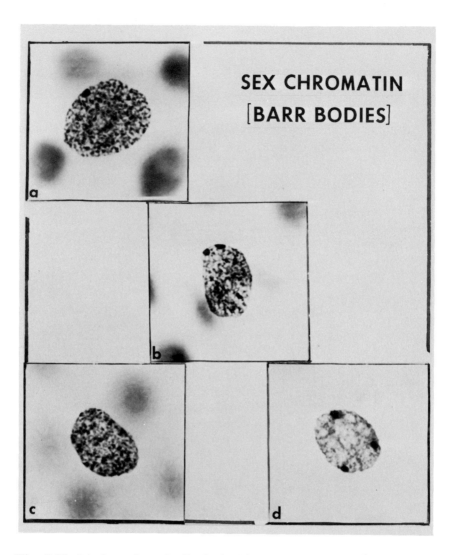

Fig. 3 Nuclei of a variety of cells obtained from the buccal mucous membrane: (a) Single Barr body; (b) Double Barr bodies; (c) No Barr body; (d) Triple Barr bodies.

A continuing study was therefore initiated in Denver in 1964, to answer two questions: 1) Can an epidemiological study of X-chromosomal non-disjunction suggest etiological factors? and 2) By comparing the frequency of non-disjunction of one of the larger chromosomes (the X) with that of a very small chromosome (Number 21) can one detect similarities in the pattern of occurrence from which one might generalize to *all* chromosomal non-disjunction?

Another purpose of this study was to identify a series of new-borns with X chromosomal anomalies in order to follow the natural course of these diseases, and in particular to evaluate their role in the later appearance of mental retardation, emotional disease, psychopathology and inadequate sexual development. Should this role be a significant one, and the data to date are highly suggestive, it will become essential to screen newborns for the presence of sex chromosomal disease in order to identify those individuals who are at risk of developing behaviorial, intellectual or sexual problems.

During the first twelve months of the study, sex chromatin determinations were carried out by means of buccal smears alone. Since then it has been found more desirable for many reasons to utilize the amniotic membrane for the sampling procedure. In any case where there was a discrepancy between the chromatin status and the phenotype of the baby, or where the phenotype suggested the possibility of Down's syndrome, the karyotype was determined.

The data has thus far been analyzed for 16,931 babies born at two neighboring Denver hospitals (A and B) with similar numbers of deliveries from January 1, 1964, until June 30, 1968. Abnormalities of the X chromosomes and of chromosomes Number 21 were scored only in babies over seven months gestation.[9]

The total number of sex chromosomal abnormalities was 26, an incidence of 0.17 percent, with that at Hospital A being 0.19 percent and at Hospital B being 0.16 percent. However, the time distribution of the aberrations is very different. During the first two years of the study, the incidence of sex chromosomal abnormalities at Hospital A was only 0.05 percent, while at Hospital B it was 0.42 percent. On the other hand, since January 1, 1966, the incidence at Hospital A has been 0.27 percent and at Hospital B, zero.

Thus far, with the exception of three babies who died in early infancy, physical and developmental examination of the affected babies have been normal.

The incidence of Trisomy 21 in the total group of newborns is 0.14 percent with the incidences at Hospital A and Hospital B being 0.19 percent and 0.07 percent respectively.

Analysis of the data revealed that 67 percent of all aberrations were born during May to October. For this reason, evidence of intra-uterine infection early in pregnancy was looked for by measuring gamma-M immunoglobulin levels in cord blood. Fifty-seven percent of 14 babies with chromosomal aberrations had gamma-M values greater than 20 mg percent whereas only 3 percent of 36 normal newborns had similar values.

Finally, an examination of the socio-economic status of affected vs. control babies suggests some skewing of the former to the lower levels.

In summary, our study thus far suggests that non-disjunction is non-random in its occurrence, that the X chromosome and Number 21 may be similarly affected, and that both intra-uterine infection and socio-economic factors may be involved in the etiology of non-disjunction.

Chromosomal disease may either involve the autosomes or the sex chromosomes. Since the organism is much more sensitive to auto-somal imbalance than to sex chromosomal imbalance, those babies born with autosomal disease are more likely to be seriously involved, being small for gestational age, and having a variety of somatic defects as well as mental retardation. These lesions are often so severe that they do not permit the birth of a viable baby. They do, however, make up the bulk of the 40 percent of spontaneous abortions which have chomosomal abnormalities. In particular, and unlike the X monosomy, autosomal monosomies with extremely rare exceptions are incompatible with the birth of a live baby.

In general, sex chromosomal disease is less severe, even though the incidence of one lesion (45,X) is 40 times more frequent among spontaneous abortions as among live births. Other individuals are less severely involved at birth, although they are likely to have mental retardation, sterility or behaviorial disturbances in later life.

It has been stated that 1 percent of newborn babies have gross chromosomal abnormalities. However, 6 percent of males and 2 percent of females in the general population show some structural abnormality of the chromosomes.[10] Hence one must be cautious in associating a chromosomal lesion etiologically with a disease. On the other hand, there would appear to be an increased incidence of these structural variants among individuals with a variety of congenital malformations (e.g. congenital heart disease and the Cornelia de Lange Syndrome), and hence it has been proposed that these familial structural chromosomal abnormalities constitute a polymorphism which predisposes to embryonic maldevelopment in genetically susceptible people.[11]

The essential utility of genetics in relation to clinical medicine is the prevention of clinical disease. This can be accomplished by genetic counseling, i.e. the prevention of the conception of individuals destined to be malformed, or by intra-uterine diagnosis of fetal disease, followed by therapeutic abortion.

Cytogenetic studies may be helpful in genetic counseling primarily by determining whether a parent's karyotype contains a structural abnormality such as a balanced translocation, which may appear in the offspring in an unbalanced form and thus produce disease. Familial Down's syndrome, for example, has been noted to occur more frequently when a parent, more commonly a mother under thirty, has a karyotype with only 45 chromosomes, one of which is abnormal, being a translocation between the long arms of two acrocentric chromosomes such as Numbers 14 and 21. Such a mother would have a risk of 20 percent with each pregnancy of having an involved child—a risk which is enormously greater than that of the average mother under 30 in the general population (0.1 percent). When the father is the carrier the average risk for each pregnancy is very much lower but still greater than normal.[5] It must be stressed that these are average figures, and it is quite possible that the translocation chromosome may segregate differently in some families. These risks must, of course, be made clear to a carrier parent seeking genetic counseling.

Examination of meiotic chromosomes obtained from testicular biopsies may be increasingly helpful in the future in establishing the presence of chromosomally unbalanced sperm in the father, even though the chromosomal lesion may not be obvious in mitotic preparations.

In recent years there has developed a new and significant branch of medicine, that of intra-uterine diagnosis. It is now possible to diagnose many genetic diseases by examination of the amniotic fluid early enough in pregnancy to permit therapeutic abortion of the diseased conceptus.

When it has been established that the pregnant woman is the carrier of a serious sex-linked recessively inherited disease (muscular dystrophy, hemophilia A, the Leche-Nyhan syndrome) a male conceptus would have a 50 percent chance of being affected whereas the female conceptus would most probably be either normal or a carrier of the genetic defect. In this case, amniocentesis would provide a sample of fetal cells whose sex chromatin status could be determined, and then, the sex of the embryo could be known by the 14th week of pregnancy. A recent report suggests that similar information may be obtained with a high degree of accuracy if as many as 1,000 mitoses obtained from culture of the peripheral blood lymphocytes of women about 14 weeks pregnant are examined.[12] The presence of a few mitoses with five G group chromosomes will indicate that the embryo is male.

In addition, fetal cells obtained from amniotic fluid can be cultivated in vitro and the karyotype of the fetus analyzed, so as to permit the diagnosis of serious chromosomal disease in time to consider therapeutic abortion. The knowledge that viruses, x-rays and certain drugs may produce significant chromosomal damage provides an additional indication for examining the fetal karyotype when the pregnant woman has been exposed to one of these agents.

Finally, these cultured cells may be subjected to biochemical tests in order to diagnose specific enzyme deficiencies characteristic of many of the inborn errors of metabolism.

Having made a diagnosis of serious fetal diseases it is now, of course, possible to abort affected embryos. The challenge and promise of the future, however, is the treatment of these diseases in utero so as to permit normal development and the birth of a normal baby.

A significant proportion of human disease, both somatic and behavioral, has a predominantly genetic etiology. The future appears bright for prevention, early diagnosis and management of these serious disorders.

REFERENCES

1. Tjio, J. H. and Levan, A.: The chromosome number of man, *Hereditas.* 42:1, 1956.

2. Puck, T. T., Cieciura, S. J. and Robinson, A.: Genetics of somatic mammalian cells. III. Long-term cultivation of euploid cells from human and animal subjects, *J. Exp. Med.* 108:945, 1958.

3. Tjio, J. H. and Whang, J.: Chromosome preparations of bone marrow cells without prior in vitro culture or in viro colchicine administration, *Stain Tech.* 37:17, 1962.

4. Tjio, J. H. and Puck, T. T.: The somatic chromosomes of man, *Proc. Nat. Acad. Sci.* 44:1229, 1959.

5. *Progress in Medical Genetics,* Vol. 6, (Arthur Steinberg and Alexander Bearn, eds). Grune and Stratton, N.Y., 1969.

6. Robinson, A.: The human chromosomes, *Am. J. Dis. Child.* 101: 379, 1961.

7. Barr, M. L. and Bertram, E. G.: A morphological distinction between neurones of the male and female, and the behavior of the nucleolar satellite during accelerated nucleoprotein synthesis, *Nature* 163:676, 1959.

8a. Lyon, M. F.: Sex chromatin and gene action in the mammalian X-chromosome, *Am. J. Hum. Genet.* 14:135, 1962.

8b. Russell, L. B.: Genetics of mammalian sex chromosomes, *Science* 133:1795, 1961.

9. Robinson, A., Goad, W. B., Puck, T. T. and Harris, J.: Studies on chromosomal non-disjunction in man. III. *Am. J. Hum. Genet.* (In Press)

10. Court Brown, W. M.: In *Human Population Genetics,* John Wiley and Sons, Inc., N.Y., 1967.

11. German, J., Ehlers, K. H., Engle, M. A.: Familial congenital heart disease. II. *Chromosomal Studies,* Circulation 34:517, 1966.

12. Walknowska, J., Conte, F. A. and Grumbach, M. M.: Practical and theoretical implications of fetal/maternal lymphocyte transfer, *Lancet* i:1116, 1969.

PRACTICAL ASPECTS OF DIETARY
REGULATION OF METABOLISM

PANEL: Drs. Goodman, Phillips, Mathias, Herman, Baker, Robinson

MODERATOR: Dr. Virginia Lee

A DISCUSSION OF ASCORBIC ACID AND
RECOMMENDED DIETARY ALLOWANCES

QUESTION: Are the recommended allowances for ascorbic acid apt to stay at the present level? What do you suggest to be the recommended dietary allowance for ascorbic acid in an adult man?

ANSWER: (Dr. Baker) There is no question that the RDA as it is today is definitely excessive. However, it has been lowered since the previous publication. The WIIO-FAO Expert Committee on Vitamins and Minerals has recently convened in Geneva and has recommended an R.I. or recommended intake of 30 milligrams per day, pretty well across the board, with the exception of an increase of 15 milligrams per day for pregnant or lactating females.

Certainly there has been adequate work, (I quote specifically the Sheffield Studies and one not too often quoted, Fox and Dangerfield's work in South Africa.) that has shown that there is no question that an intake of around 10 milligrams is perfectly adequate to cure scurvy. You want to consider this, then, as a so-called "minimal intake." Any level that is recommended beyond this becomes merely a pontifical question because there is no body of data to give good evidence as to whether any N milligram excess is going to enhance ascorbate metabolism for the well-being of the individual. Certainly the 30 milligram level is being recommended by WHO. It was arrived at by simply taking what one might consider as a minimal intake plus two standard deviations. Once again, this is the business of attempting to satiate 97½ percent of the population. If you want to add another standard deviation, then you can go to 102 percent of the population, but I don't think this is necessary at this time.

QUESTION: There were a couple of questions directed to the possibility that the high dietary Vitamin C intake is responsible for hyper-cholesterolemia in the U.S. population.

ANSWER: (Dr. Baker) I don't think that we have sufficient evidence at this time to say that it is or that it is not. Certainly, from what was seen of the effect upon cholesterol levels in the Iowa City Study, one would have to say that the higher the level of intake of ascorbic acid, apparently the higher the level of the blood cholesterol. Now this does not intimate a metabolic cause or effect. Before anyone could make any recommendations or statements, we would have to have much more data in this area because here we are dealing with what would be a regulatory mechanism.

ANSWER: (Dr. Herman) The problem about cholesterol is that it is true that atherosclerotic plagne have cholesterol in them. This has been known for a hundred years or so, and it is possible to produce lesions in animals that resemble human atherosclerosis by feeding cholesterol, and it is true that very high levels of cholesterol in the blood presuppose atherosclerosis. Those are the facts. Now whether a given level of cholesterol in a particular individual will lead to coronary artery disease is completely unknown. Whether one can regulate the level of cholesterol in the blood by dietary cholesterol restriction is not clear because the body makes cholesterol, so if you don't eat cholesterol the body makes it, and the mechanisms that control the blood level of cholesterol are poorly understood.

What really is important with coronary artery disease is whether or not the lesions develop in the blood vessel, and not really what is in the blood. So it is possible to have high blood cholesterol and never have any coronary artery disease. It is also possible to have coronary artery disease with normal or low levels of cholesterol. So there are many factors involved in coronary artery disease, and nobody understands really why a particular level of cholesterol occurs in any individual. I would think from many lines of evidence that the level in man is probably more on a genetic basis than any dietary basis, though it is possible to control levels of cholesterol by a number of dietary maneuvers or administration of a variety of drugs. Certainly the people who have hypercholesterolemia on a familial or genetic basis, the so-called Type Two hyper-lypoproteinemia, certainly this is unrelated to ascorbic acid intake.

QUESTION: (to Dr. Goodman) If a woman is unsuccessful in breast-feeding and her baby gains only one pound during the first six weeks of life after coming home from the hospital, has this baby had enough protein to promote normal brain growth? (At six weeks of age the baby was put on Similac.)

ANSWER: (Dr. Goodman) I don't know, and I doubt if anyone really does know, since in the course of development in the human brain there is relatively little known as to what is made when, what the reserves of the child are to be drawn upon, etc. So I really don't know.

QUESTION: What effect did your experiments have on the number or ratio of neuron and other cells in the brain and how would you predict such changes, if you have them, would affect learning or memory?

ANSWER: (Dr. Goodman) We don't know. All we know, and all anybody has measured thus far in the brain of these animals, is the total amount of DNA. Now it has been said here a couple of times, and it most probably is true, that there are more and more cell types being found in the brain in which the number of chromosomes is doubled or more. In other words, that you have more DNA in some cells of the brain than you have in other cells. If this is true, then this hypothesis that changes in DNA are directly related to a change in cell number may not be true, and one always has to keep this in the back of the mind. So I don't feel free in saying that because we get a decrease of 10 percent in these newborn brains, they have 10 percent less cells. That may not be the case.

Now as to whether these are neurons *or* glia or neurons *and* glia, nobody knows. This type of approach is new; my own entry into the field is very new; the people who go in, go in from a prejudiced point of view. They are either psychologists, or they are DNA chemists or this sort of thing. We don't always have the technology immediately available to do these sorts of things. It is not the kind of thing you just sit down and do, start counting glia and neurons. It takes a good deal of tooling up, a good deal of training, etc. The truth of the matter is, nobody has done it. Now in time this is one of the things we have in mind which we want to look at, but there is always this problem that there are so many things you want to do—which do you do first? So the answer to the question is—we don't know.

Assuming that there are less cells, we don't know whether it is neurons or glia. If one had to take a guess with the knowledge we have presently, one would guess it is predominantly neurons, but that may be erroneous. All I am saying is there is a need for much more research along this line. Now let us assume that it is neurons or glia or a mixture, but a decrease in cell number. Does this have implications in learning and memory? The answer to that question is also my standard, I don't know, because I don't understand the mechanisms of learning and memory, I don't understand what the glia cell does in the nervous system; I don't even understand what the neuron does, and I think the answer to that question is some distance away. We must learn a great deal more about basic function of some of these things in the nervous system before we can really say a decrease in neurons would affect this. It would depend which neurons; a decrease in one set of neurons may have an effect on learning and memory, a decrease in another set may have no effect on this. The answers I have for all my students on these questions are I don't know, nobody knows, or I don't know *if* anybody knows.

QUESTION: Quite a few questions came up after Dr. Robinson's talk. One of them is: Many people are concerned with the effect of sugar substitutes used over a period of time, particularly since recent research with mice has produced defects in their genes. What is your opinion?

ANSWER: (Dr. Robinson) I presume the question refers to the statement that chromosomal breaks can result from some of these food additives. The problem of whether or not a specific substance working in vivo actually produces an increased number of chromosomal breaks is a very difficult one to determine. The reason is there are whole varieties of things that can produce chromosomal breaks, so that in order to know whether this specific substitute does cause chromosomal breaks, one has to know in detail the past history of the person whose chromosomes we are checking. So that if, for example, he is exposed to a hepatitis virus or a measles virus or possibly even a cold virus prior to the time that you are looking at his chromosomes, his increased number of breaks could be due to the past history, to the exposure he has had to x-ray or some such thing, or to many, many other factors that we are not aware of which can produce chromosomal breaks.

But an even more important question is, what is the significance of a chromosomal break if it occurs? We don't know that. We do know that there are many more breaks which tend to heal, presumably normally, that we don't see. We know this from the fact that if we take cells and expose them to doses of x-rays and then look at the chromosomes at varying periods of time after exposure, the number of breaks that one sees goes down very rapidly because re-healing has occurred.

You realize, of course, that chromosome is gross anatomy. There are thousands of genes on each chromosome, and parenthetically I might state that I get many requests for chromosomal analysis on patients who have molecular disease, who have inborn errors of metabolism. Our microscopes aren't that good. You can't see a molecule under a microscope. So a molecular disease won't show up with a chromosomal aberration. Similarly, when these gross structures re-heal, have they re-healed on a molecular level or are they, in fact, point mutations which are molecular, biochemical changes? Have they occurred and are we not aware of them? We don't know the answer to that.

So 1) we don't know the significance of these chromosomal breaks; 2) the food additives, whether or not they produce breaks in humans, we don't know. The evidence is in mice, and mice are like humans in many ways, but also unlike them in many respects; 3) the dosages which are used for these particular experiments are very different from the levels of the substances which are present in the tissues in an individual taking food additives. All we can say about that, like we say about everything else, is we view with alarm, and that is as much as we can say. Of course, this whole problem has been much more carefully examined in regard to some of the drugs, particularly LSD. Even there, where it has been very carefully examined, where patients have been used as their own controls, still the answer is indefinite. But there is enough there for us to view with alarm.

QUESTION: What is the cost of the chromosome screening test such as you conducted with the newborn?

ANSWER: (Dr. Robinson) The test with the newborn is quite reasonable. We will do twenty to forty of those in a day, and roughly it would be somewhere between $2.00 and $5.00 per examination.

QUESTION: (to Dr. Herman) Since lactose enhances calcium absorption in the gut, is there any indication that calcium deficiency is prevalent in lactase deficiency?

ANSWER: (Dr. Herman) No, in the patients that we have seen with lactase deficiency, there really isn't any calcium deficiency. The calcium in the milk or milk products is absorbed normally despite the fact that there is a lactase deficiency. In a large number of individuals who have been studied with lactase deficiency there has been no evidence of calcium deficiency or any type of rickets or osteoporosis that develops or osteomalacia.

QUESTION: There are several questions to Dr. Herman with respect to carbohydrate diets. The first is, what type of carbohydrate should a "normal" individual try to include in his diet?

ANSWER: (Dr. Herman) Certainly any kind of carbohydrate that causes any type of symptom should be eliminated from the diet. We see many patients who have symptoms because of carbohydrate intolerance. Some of this carbohydrate intolerance causes symptoms because some of the individuals have reactive hypoglycemia. That is, they have an increased output of insulin because of the increased input of glucose, and this insulin output is higher than it ought to be; it is out of syncrony, out of phase with the rise in blood glucose. So as a consequence, a secondary hypoglycemia develops, and the individual develops symptoms. So in these types of individuals, carbohydrates in general, generally glucose containing substances which would mean most carbohydrate in the diet, should be eliminated.

We have other patients whose problems are not quite so simple who get considerable difficulty and discomfort with carbohydrates, and it is not clear what the nature of their disease is. Some of these people do not adapt their enzymes in the jejunum as the normal individuals do, so we think there is some connection; that is, the lack of adaption to carbohydrates leads to symptoms in some way and these individuals we generally advise to eliminate carbohydrates from their diet. So if carbohydrate causes any kind of symptom, and you must be sure that this is the case, then it must be eliminated.

In the case of the normal individual, there are epidemiologic studies to suggest that sucrose is associated with a higher incidence of coronary artery disease or other atherosclerotic type diseases. It is possible there is a sub-population of people in the total population who tolerate sucrose not as well as others. This seems to be related to fructose. It has been well demonstrated now from our work and from other people's work that fructose is metabolized by man at a very rapid rate to fatty acids to form triglyceride, so that in the blood you can elevate serum triglycerides with fructose or fructose containing sugar, sucrose for example, in man as well as in animals.

It seems that there is some relationship of a high sucrose intake to a coronary artery disease. Now this may not be true for everybody, and this may be only one factor, so we are at the present postulating, or have a working hypothesis that sucrose is not the best type of sugar for individauls. Now we all know that there is a high incidence of dental disease with a high sucrose intake, and the people who avoid all sugars, such as certain people who are intolerant to fructose and have what is called a central fructosaria (this is a rare disease), learn very quickly that anything sweet is associated with very uncomfortable symptoms or very severe disease. So they avoid all sugar. These people have a very low incidence of dental disease, very little dental caries. So sucrose is bad for teeth; it seems to raise blood triglycerides when taken to excess, and maybe some people are more snsitive than others.

There are other patients who have what is called carbohydrate-induced hyperlipemia. These are people who with any kind of carbohydrate have very high levels of blood triglycerides with associated elevated blood cholesterol. These people probably should not be on a high carbohydrate diet, and the therapeutic measures in these people are sometimes rather complicated. There is a variety of dietary things that one does, a variety of drugs. These people have no symptoms, but they have elevated blood lipids, and they have a higher incidence in many cases, in many of these types of diseases, of atherosclerosis.

So, as a general rule, we have to say that not everybody can eat everything. Those who get symptoms related to reactive hypoglycemia or other gastro-intestinal symptoms, should not eat a high carbohydrate diet; those who have specific deficiencies such as lactase, sucrase, or maltase, should avoid those specific sugars or the dietary sources; those who have the various types of hyperlipemia, particularly the carbohydrate or hyperlipoproteinemia, should avoid high carbohydrate diet. And then probably in general, sucrose should be avoided since too much of it will cause dental troubles, and this is a very serious problem.

There is a tremendous amount of dental disease in the population which is a very tremendous economic drain, and also there is the suggestion that it is related epidimeologically to atherosclerosis. You have to eat some carbohydrate, so a moderate carbohydrate diet, probably not sucrose, is what we would recommend at the moment for the average individual who has no specific disease. But not all disease related to carbohydrate is necessarily symptomatic. Now that is a complicated answer, I know. It merely points out that the problem we are dealing with doesn't have simple answers which everybody would like to have, but it is complicated. So, we must individualize rather than making sweeping statements which can apply to populations entirely.

ANSWER: (Dr. Phillips) Back to potatoes. I wanted to add one remark to Dr. Herman's comment on the importance or potential importance of fructose in coronary disease. Probably one of the biggest dietary changes that we have from our fathers and grandfathers in the development and the increasing incidence of coronary heart disease is that we take in a greater portion of our carbohydrate diet as sucrose and fructose, instead of as starches as they did. This increased production of fatty acids and glucogenesis from fructose may be what is contributing to our increase in cardiac disease in this population as compared to our predecessors. They ate a high starch diet from carbohydrates where we tend to be more on a high sucrose and fructose diet.

QUESTION: (to Dr. Mathias) What implications do your studies have on the type and amounts of fat to be included in diets for "normal" people?

ANSWER: (Dr. Mathias) You remember some of the control mechanisms that I talked about—Dr. Herman's group has very beautifully shown, as well as others, that actually what happens when you are feeding the fructose molecule is you've by-passed one of the controlling enzymes that I talked about, PFK enzyme. So you get a tremendous amount of acetate, and it is built up as fatty acids. That is the only place you can put it. It is a one-way system. So, instead of talking about the amount of fat we can feed (we can feed carbohydrate and it is going to end up as fat, too) let's talk about the type of fat.

That is what my answer would be to that question—it is not how much fat or how much carbohydrate that matters, because in the cell they are going to end up as saturated fat, and that is what we are going to store, no matter how many calories of each we eat. However, dietarily we can control the kind of fat because we also have the alternative of feeding polyunsaturated fat which fructose cannot be converted into, the polyunsaturated type. These are metabolized much faster than the saturated type, so we get into metabolic adaptations. Probably what happens, which Dr. Dupont has shown, is that when you are feeding polyunsaturates they are catabolized faster and you end up with less carbons being able to store in the adipose tissue and it is just burned up as CO_2.

QUESTION: This question has to do with starvation diets and protein. In starvation, patients are in negative nitrogen-balance. When this is continued over a long period, what assurance is there that there is not breakdown of tissue of vital organs which in the long run may be deleterious to the starved individual's health? [The questioner goes on to relate that a recent diet book is based on a very low protein intake, and that protein allowed is incomplete protein. The purpose of this diet is to get rid of unsightly bulges left after regular weight reduction.]

ANSWER: (Dr. Herman) We have a problem in the United States where we have people who have access to as much food as they want. People do things when it is pleasant, and they avoid things when it is painful. Some people have appetites which they cannot control—it is very painful to be hungry. So these people eat, whether you want to call it a neurotic state, a compulsive eater type syndrome akin to other compulsive types of activity or not, or whether you want to say there is a psychologic dependence, or whether you want to say there is biochemical abnormality which doesn't permit them to regulate their appetite. The fact is they do eat to excess and they have access to all the food they want.

We see many people who are enormously overweight. We had one patient who weighed 489 pounds, and his weight probably should have been no more than 200 at the most. You are faced with the problem in these people of how to reduce them. One way is to put them on a low caloric intake. The problem comes that it takes a very long time. Nobody gets overweight overnight. If you gain a half a pound a week, in a year you only gain 25 pounds. If you get a hundred pounds overweight, at that rate, it still takes four years. If you were to lose a pound a week, you'd only lose 50 pounds in a year on the average; it takes two years to lose 100 pounds, and most people are unwilling or unable to persist with diets for that period of time.

So many people (the massively overweight individual who is unable to refrain from taking in food to excess), are put on a starvation diet as another approach. You lose about a pound of weight a day. That means you can reduce people very rapidly compared to a low calorie diet. There are some problems of weight fluctuations with the water retention or water loss, but on the average one loses about a pound a day.

Now of course, when you do reduce individuals this way, they lose fat, but they also lose nitrogen. It is true they go into a negative nitrogen balance. They also go into a negative potassium, a negative sodium balance; they go into a negative balance in everything because they are taking in nothing and they are losing everything. We generally allow them access to water and vitamins, and people seem to tolerate this fairly well, particularly when they are all by themselves. They don't see anybody eating, don't smell food, and they become acidotic, so they lose the stimulus to appetite, the stimulus for taking in food.

Now there have been reports of people on very long fasts, several hundred days or a half a year, six months. And with occasional sugar supplementation or something of this sort. Occasionally an individual has become so acidiotic that he becomes very ill and in some cases has died suddenly. There is a recent report in the journal *Lancet* where an individual on a six or nine month fast because of massive obesity died suddenly during the refeeding period. The heart showed fragmented myocardial fibrosis. There was a large argument in the "Letters to the Editor" following that report as to what the nature of the microscopic findings in the heart were. We see other people who are being fasted who develop a high blood uric acid. This almost invariably happens. Some of these individuals develop joint pains—it looks like gout, a secondary type of gout.

So the problem comes, when you fast people totally, what should you replete them with? We have done some studies where we have measured glucose tolerance tests, and almost everybody who fasts develops an abnormal glucose tolerance test. This can be prevented in part by repleting with potassium. The question comes, can you prevent any muscle loss if you give a small amount of protein? What I would be afraid of is that the protein itself is toxic. If you give protein at very high levels it can be toxic because, remember, protein de-animates to ammonia, which is a very toxic material, and there have to be mechanisms for eliminating it.

Consequently, the answer to what you give fasting people is not known. What would have to be studied would be fasting people with various kinds of intakes, either very low carbohydrate or very low carbohydrate low protein, or perhaps mineral supplementation—things of this sort. If I gave somebody no fat, no carbohydrate, just amino acids, I am afraid they would get much sicker than they might become if they had a total fast. There have been a lot of studies done on starving people, and it has been shown that if you keep the people quiet, give them access to water, they can starve for as long as six months. Then you can refeed them. It is true, they do go into negative nitrogen balance, and they do lose some muscle mass; but nobody has been able to figure out how to lose fat and not nitrogen. There doesn't seem to be any way to do this, and the minute you give any other caloric intake, you immediately slow down the weight losing process.

Starvation is an extremely complicated phenomenon, and those people who have studied it in far greater detail propose the idea that man used to be a hunter, and the mechanisms in the body have been developed so that he would be able to kill, eat, gorge himself, and then rest for several days, and be able to withstand fasting until he could find an animal that he could kill and eat again. Our modern civilization has negated what our biochemistry was built to withstand.

QUESTION: (to Dr. Robinson) Are all mongoloids the product of a chromosome anomoly?

ANSWER: (Dr. Robinson) When I went to medical school, *always* and *never* were two words that I was always told never to say. So I can't answer that, but I would say that the vast, vast majority of children with Down's syndrome (and I prefer that term to mongolism because this has nothing to do with the Oriental race. The name came because a British pediatrician didn't like Orientals), the vast majority have chromosomal abnormality. Now there have been some children reported who had all of the clinical stigmata of Down's syndrome who did not have the chromosomal lesion. They are very rare. These may be the individuals who are the mosaics that I talked about, who may have had two or more populations of cells, some of which were normal in their chromosomal constitution and some abnormal. Or they may have been chromosomes where translocation had occurred—translocation with such a small piece of chromosome, but a vital piece, that it couldn't be picked up under the microscope. But the answer is that 99.9 percent of all children with Down's do have a chromosomal malformation.

QUESTION: Has any research been done in relation to the age of the sperm and the incidence of Down's syndrome?

ANSWER: (Dr. Robinson) As the person who asked that question probably knows, there is what we call the maternal effect in the incidence of Down't syndrome. That is that older mothers, and by older in this context we mean mothers primarily over 35 years of age at the time of conception, have a much higher risk of having non-disjunction occur and particularly non-disjunction involving Chromosome Number 21 which produces Down's syndrome. There seems to be no relationship between paternal age and the occurrence of non-disjunction. Paternal age means the age of the father, not necessarily the age of the sperm. The sperm, unlike the ovum, is different in its origins.

A man in the fertile period of his life produces a new population of sperm roughly every two months, whereas a female is born with all the ova that she is ever going to have. Therefore, when she conceives at the age of 35 or 40, the ovum involved in that fertilization is 35 or 40 years old, and perhaps it is a little rusty; perhaps that is why non-disjunction is more likely to occur. But you see in man that doesn't occur, because man doesn't produce sperm until he enters puberty, and then after that he has a new population coming up roughly every 60 to 90 days.

QUESTION: (to Dr. Phillips) What is the real practical significance for the practicing dietitian of all the steps in the metabolism of glucose and amino acid? Why should she bother about trying to understand it, or should she?

ANSWER: (Dr. Phillips) I like Dr. Goodman's answer — I don't know. I don't think that a practicing dietitian would have to be familiar with each and every step of glycolysis and lipid synthesis and lipid degradation, but I do think that a basic understanding of the flow of metabolites through the metabolic pathways is of value. I think that it helps to know that carbohydrate can be converted into fats and that amino acids enter into the same metabolic scheme and can be converted back into carbohydrates; that this is what occurs in an individual who is fasting. That is why you are getting a breakdown of proteins as Dr. Herman mentioned; that the protein is being degraded and that a good share of the amino acids are being converted into glucose, and that this ocurs in the liver. But as far as remembering that it goes from this compound to that compound by such and such an enzyme, and that you need this co-factor or that co-factor, I don't think that is probably essential information for a practicing dietitian, but I would feel that a broad knowledge of this flow of metabolites is of a great deal of importance.

ANSWER: (Dr. Herman) This problem is not unique to dietitians. My nurses ask me this; medical students ask me this; even the interns and residents in the medical wards ask me this. They say we can practice medicine without knowing biochemistry. That is true. You can also practice medicine without a license or ever going to school, and I daresay that most of the public might not ever know that, except for the law, when you are caught without a diploma. We usually tell medical students, you have to learn biochemistry because if you fail you can be thrown out of medical school, and so if you want to go on to the second year, you had better pass the first.

The point is that dietetics and nutrition is really a part of biochemistry because foods are chemicals. They just taste good. The usual chemicals in the laboratory taste rotten, but food tastes good, and it is a very complicated mixture of chemicals; it is very important to know how they are disposed. I agree that you should know the overall pathways, what happens to them, and what things go wrong, not that you know the kinetics of every enzyme or the amino acid structure or the current theory of how enzymes work. But you should know how these things are disposed, what happens to them, so that you can interpret your own literature intelligently and know what is important and what is not. You don't know all the details, but you should know what foods people should eat and why they have to eat them, what can go wrong in a general sense. The important thing that you are asking is, do I memorize all the pathways? All the enzymes? The answer is *no*. You should *learn* them.

QUESTION: (to Dr. Baker) Please comment on the ethics and morality of depleting a human's body of ascorbic acid. Do you believe that in the Iowa City Studies the escape of the two prisoner volunteers was related to the stress they were undergoing during the clinical trials?

ANSWER: (Dr. Baker) Absolutely not. In fact it was a very simple problem that they didn't like our hospitality. They probably would have still been on the ward if they hadn't liberated certain articles of value from the University Club and decided that they had better leave our care. This shouldn't be taken jokingly, because any time you run a depletion-repletion study, certainly you are going to have some psychological problems with your subjects in the depleted stage.

To be specific, we have seen this in both scurvy studies. Once you tell a man that he is receiving all food, essential foods, with the exception of a particular essential micro-nutrient or macro-nutrient, you can be self-assured that he can dream up all kinds of symptoms, and as the deficiency state proceeds, his can become an exaggerated problem. Actually we were fairly lucky in having just two depart, because there are a couple of things here that are even worse than deficiency. That diet was a corn oil-casein-safflower oil-vitamin and mineral mix. It was not taken orally. They took it by pumping it down with a naso-gastric tube. Now if you had a diet like this for a period of approximately five months, I am sure you would become quite unhappy with it.

Insofar as the stress is concerned, I said nothing this morning, but interestingly enough, at the peak of deficiency the four subjects were surgically wounded by an incision on the thigh; punch biopsies were taken of the healing tissue once a week. We were not able to show any difference in the rate of catabolism, nor could we show any increase in the rate of catabolism; nor could we show any increased presence of any of the isotopically labeled material within the tissue. We did, however, have one subject who underwent severe emotional stress. There is no need going into detail.

I think you will find this in the *Journal of Medical Nutrition* in the May issue—that the catabolic rate did in fact double, that here would be a serious question as to whether that increase in rate was due to the drug which he was treated with or to the emotional state that he was suffering from.

QUESTION: (to Dr. Robinson) Would you comment on the theory that a virus is a gene gone wild?

ANSWER: (Dr. Robinson) A virus, of course, is a very simple bit of organic material which contains either DNA or RNA which is, as you know, genetically very important, plus a protein coat. The virus cannot live outside of a cellular environment, can't multiply outside of a cellular environment, so it is a parasite. Now it is known that particularly in bacteria, certain ones called phages can infect the bacterium and then the DNA or RNA can become part of the genetic material of the infected bacterium. The certain viruses can also infect bacteria, pick up some of the genetic material from a given bacteria, and then when it leave that bacterium convey that genetic material to another bacterium, so that you get what is known as transduction — genes taken from one type of organism into another with the virus being the vector. So that a virus does have genes in it and those genes can, at least in very simple organisms, change the genetic material of those organisms. If that can be defined as a gene going wild, I suppose it is a gene gone wild. It is possible to change the genetic material of simple organisms by viral infection.

QUESTION: If there is a possibility of second generation effect of inadequate quality or quantity of prenatal diets, could that have implications for breaking the poverty cycle where grandparents, parents, and children eventually get on relief roles?

ANSWER: (Dr. Goodman) It is a perplexing question, and it is a loaded question, because you say is there a possibility? Yes, there is a possibility. The question is, is there a probability? I might cite some interesting experiments which lead me to a little insight into this, which are in the literature. One is a group of hypo-pituitary mice which have less DNA in their brains than norm.al mice. You can super-feed these animals and get them to grow, and you can do this in the immediate postnatal period. The body grows, but the brain does not. Now if we go to the things that I talked about in the rat where you put three pups on a mother rather than twelve, in that case both the brain size and the brain DNA were increased above normal. The only difference here, if we can go across species for a minute, is that this is a hypo-pituitary animal and the speculation is that there is something in the brain of the normal animal, in the development of the hypothalamus and the pituitary of the normal animal, which controls part of the brain growth.

If one could go one step further to speculate, I can go to one other experiment which was Aminol's work a couple of years ago, in which he gave a mother during the gestation period, a period of about two weeks I believe, growth hormone, bovine growth hormone. The newborn of these mothers had increased brain DNA over normal rats, but the animal size was not increased. So this is the other side of the coin. If one can speculate, and one can speculate, that the maternal environment—the hypothalamus pituitary of the mother—can in some way affect the development of the hypothalamus and pituitary of her offspring so that it does not develop, then this thing will be carried on and on and on. Once that section does not develop properly, then it, in itself, in each generation would not develop. That is *pure* speculation; that is *wild* speculation. But there is such a possibility.

Now it is another question as to what poverty is all about, and the poverty cycle. The fact that a certain portion of the brain might not develop and you might end up with smaller individuals, etc., etc., since generally small brain size is associated with a smaller individual, statistically speaking, this says nothing about the mental ability, the drive, etc., of this person. We have to be very careful that we don't confuse these issues, that if there is more or less DNA, we have a smarter or a less smart animal, person, etc. That would be a very dangerous mistake, and I could say yes, there is a possibility that there are second generation defects. This needs a great deal of work, and it will be forthcoming, I am sure, but all we can do at this point is keep an open mind. I think I will leave it at that.

QUESTION: Nutritional status studies reveal inadequate dietary intakes of cirtus fruits and milks in population groups. It appears that nutritionists should re-evaluate nutrition education programs to increase ascorbic acid intake on the basis of Scurvy I and II Studies and milk in adults and certain ethnic groups.

ANSWER: (Dr. Herman) I think the only comment I shall make is that it should be realized that not all dietary substances are for all people, and that sometimes we can detect individuals with very gross difficulties and sometimes we suspect that there are very subtle problems related to dietary intake. I see this particularly when I see patients who have all sorts of obscure problems and symptoms, and we try to determine what the nature of the disease is. Often these people have been seen by numbers of physicians, have finally been sent to the psychiatrist. The patient gets discouraged and the doctor gets frustrated, and in some of these people, particularly those who have some sort of gastro-intestinal symptoms and have been told that they have a nervous stomach or some other emotional disturbance leading to gastro-intestinal disturbance—we should recognize that very subtle problems with regard to dietary intake can cause difficulty.

I suspect that there are people who do have lactase deficiency of a mild nature that causes some difficulties sometimes, some bloating, some uncomfortably full feeling after they drink milk or take something that has a lot of lactose in it. All this points up is that this is one element that can cause people difficulty. I am sure there must be others that we just don't ordinarily recognize. Not every person with symptoms or problems goes to see a doctor. We see a lot of people with headaches, for example, just to pick a very common symptom that women often have. There are fifty or sixty different causes of headaches, some of which we know, some are serious, some are trivial. Oftentimes we have people with headaches that we never find a cause for; we only give temporary relief with medication.

Is any of this related to any of the environmental things they come in contact with? High altitude before they are acclimatized? Certain dietary constituents, various kinds of drugs, the humidity, the heat, all sorts of environmental changes? Diet is just one of many environmental substances that has an influence and can be very subtle, and milk is only one particular example. I think people don't always know what should or shouldn't be eaten — they are not always able to relate symptoms to their dietary intake. So with regard to milk, all I can say is until we know really from screening populations who has lactase deficiency and to what degree, it is hard to say who should or shouldn't take in milk. There is no easy screening method, really, and we have to leave it up to the individual.

I suspect sometimes when children don't want to drink their milk, maybe they do get uncomfortable and they don't want to complain. Maybe they find that if they do complain of symptoms, their parents are unsympathetic. Their parents have learned that milk is a perfect food, and every child should have it; every growing child should have it. If the kid doesn't want to drink it he is being stubborn or ornery, yet maybe he does have symptoms, maybe he is uncomfortable and just doesn't appreciate it.

We see a lot of adults, for example, who have been having so-called nervous diarrhea or nervous gastro-intestinal disorder. It turns out very simply they have lactase deficiency. Everybody is very much relieved because here is an organic defect and it isn't all in the mind after all. Perhaps we have a lot of subtle things of this sort, and perhaps we should just keep an open mind. When we don't know, we should admit we don't know and not try to make a diagnosis or decide what a person should or shouldn't eat. We should get direct information, but this is not always easy to get.

ANSWER: (Dr. Baker) I don't want to push the citrus industry one way or the other because I enjoy citrus fruit myself. Certainly in terms of dietary education we can't say that C is a problem because scurvy is not something that is prominent today as it was years ago — although, in fact, it still exists. Much of it exists because of dietary fadism, because of inadequate education. One interesting facet is this: in attempting to prepare a so-called solid diet for the Iowa City subjects, we found that it was absolutely impossible to prepare any normal diet, no matter how long it was boiled, how long it was autoclaved, that contained less than three milligrams of C in the daily ration. Certainly that is not going to be adequate.

But by the same token, at the same time we were trying to produce scurvy in our volunteers, the attending physician's secretary had been going from physician to physician with some rather odd skin disease that seemed to defy all diagnosis and all treatment. After a number of differing physicians and heaven knows how many differing treatments, someone finally decided to run a blood Vitamin C on her, and lo and behold there was no Vitamin C. In checking out over the dietary history, it became quite obvious that here was a forty-two year old lady who was attempting to maintain a twenty-year-old figure and in order to do it she had two pieces of dry toast and tea in the morning for breakfast. Well, there is no C in that, I can assure you, only a trace. She ate one hamburger without too much dressing on it and a glass of milk for lunch. There is very little C in milk, and essentially none in hamburger. There is, by the way, in hot dogs, remember. The supper would consist of a piece of broiled meat, no vegetable and again, dry bread. This had gone on for a period of eighteen months; that is how long it took her to produce signs and symptoms which by the way, if you are curious, were totally cured by the administration of 50 milligrams of C per day for a period of five days.

So, it is real, and it can occur, and there is an educational process. Now as to anything beyond a reasonable intake, my point of view is about the same as that of the British. About the only thing that it is good for is cleaning the copper drains, because it will be excreted unchanged.

IV

NUTRITION IN HUMAN
ECOLOGY AND CULTURE

GEOGRAPHIC DIMENSIONS OF HUMAN ECOLOGY

HORACE F. QUICK
Department of Geography
University of Colorado
Boulder, Colorado

Human ecology once had a geography. Before the advent of closed environmental systems, which is not at all long ago, the human being was part of a natural environment or ecosystem.

The geography of man is, of course, now very much homogenized as a result of communication and transport in particular. There was a time, however, and less than a few thousand years ago, when different kinds of men were part of a definite ecosystem and there were earthly environments where there were no men at all.

If one examines a modern map of world population, two preliminary observations can be made immediately. Mankind seems to be concentrated in a distribution pattern through the present equatorial regions of Earth, and the polar regions are shown as entirely uninhabited. Human beings are dependent upon primary and secondary producers in a complicated food chain, and therefore a whole biotic complex must have some pattern of distribution. This pattern leads one to postulate a "First Approximation of Biotic Distribution."

In a fashion of geographic analysis one may proceed to relate the earth's present heat belt, the equatorial regions, with a higher level of primary production, or to search for some other environmental factor or combination of factors favorable to the human race.

Much emphasis has been placed, of recent years, on estimates of biological productivity. This "productivity" has an important significance for mankind in that it includes among other things the supply of nutrition for human life.

Other environmental factors are at work, however, that affect the density of human population as well as distribution. The basic biologic capacity to reproduce appears to be the same among all human beings regardless of race or geographic residence. Controls on population density then must be environmental, or cultural, or coactions of environment and culture. Life is hazardous for all but appears to be more so for arctic peoples who never seem to have been able to achieve that glorious mark of civilization known as the "population explosion."

We conventionally think of the necessities of life as food, water and shelter. Human physiology, as it has evolved over the millenia, has drawn for more of human history on the productivity of a natural environment than upon the modified environment of the so-called technological age. We further note the conventional order in which we commonly think of the necessities of life, food being first mentioned.

It follows very simply that man's environment has always provided his needs or we should not be there today. But there is a geographic dimension to food production which has a bearing on the fortunes of population and so we find a primordial geography of nutrition related to the geography of man.

Polar regions have a very low, indeed are nearly devoid of, edible green plant production. We may think of Eskimos, Samoyedes and other arctic tribes of men as having evolved on a non-plant diet or adapted to it. In contrast, we may think of the denser populations of tropic and sub-tropic regions as having evolved on the abundant plant productivity of their heat-belt environments.

So much for a generalized introduction to the subject of geographic dimensions of human ecology, and for an evasion of definitions. The problem of the chicken and the egg has perplexed us for a long time but most thinking people would agree that an environment of some kind had to exist before people could exist.

Out of this simple thought a simple model can be constructed to show the fundamental structure of human ecology. It contains three factor-groups commonly known as Environment, Population and Culture. Given the existence of Environment before a population could exist, the model can be begun as

ENVIRONMENT → POPULATION

where the two terms are understood and the symbol borrowed from the chemist means "yields."

Ecologists busy themselves describing environmental changes both temporal and locational. Places on earth have not always been what they are today and this evolution of environment can be expressed most simply with sub-script numbers, $E_1 \rightarrow E_2$ meaning environmental change in time and place.

Having agreed that population is dependent upon an environment, we add the POPULATION group of factors as P_1, to indicate a primitive population in a natural environment, E_1.

$$E_1 \rightarrow P_1$$

Evolution over periods of time can be indicated with subscript numbers to show a succession of developmental stages. The development of a culture can be added as the symbol C, embracing a complex of cultural factors or characteristics as shown in Figure 1.

At the subsistence level of development, the impact of population on environment is neglible and natural ecologic restoration keeps pace with resource exploitation. In later stages, people might have begun modifying their environment and it seems most logical that the first cultural modification would concern food production or the techniques of obtaining food.

This last step in a model simulation of the EPC relationship produces what we might call the outline of human ecology.

The manifestations of cultural impact on environment are all too numerous but one of particular interest in the context of this symposium concerns the modification of environment in terms of shelter, clothing and activity which bear on the nutritional demands of modern man.

A reduction of physical activity might be leading to a form of "undernourishment" manifesting lower body weights of youth and ultimately of the population. Some might lay the blame on the age of the wheel, but regardless of cause, articles are beginning to appear in the literature that describe the undernourishment of people in the face of food surpluses. We are also seeing over-nourishment resulting in heart disease and other debilities. Outside of this feed-back effect

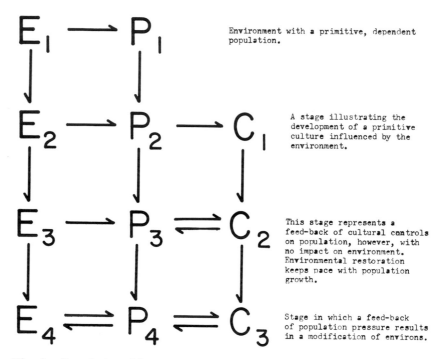

$E_1 \longrightarrow E_2$ Illustrating environmental change over a period of time; the subscript numerals refer to a sequence of time periods.

$E_1 \longrightarrow P_1$ Environment with a primitive, dependent population.

$E_2 \longrightarrow P_2 \longrightarrow C_1$ A stage illustrating the development of a primitive culture influenced by the environment.

$E_3 \longrightarrow P_3 \rightleftharpoons C_2$ This stage represents a feed-back of cultural controls on population, however, with no impact on environment. Environmental restoration keeps pace with population growth.

$E_4 \rightleftharpoons P_4 \rightleftharpoons C_3$ Stage in which a feed-back of population pressure results in a modification of environs.

Fig. 1. Foundation of human ecology: environment-population-culture model.

of the age of technology resulting from a combination of social-cultural impact on environment, there still exist some rather unaltered ecological conditions under which some people live. These provide a datum or reference point against which we may evaluate the present status of human ecology and its evolution. These environments yield quite different natural products as sources of nutrition for the people indigenous to the regions. From the simple facts of geography it is easy to conclude that the nutritional needs of the indigenes must closely approximate the demands of the environment. Otherwise, no human population would exist there.

For the purpose of illustration, a generalization could be stated that arctic peoples survive and maintain good health on a diet of meat, both lean and fat, for there is practically no edible plant production there. Tropical peoples have a very low fat and meat demand. The two environments make grossly different demands on the indigenous people. Some populations of polar and equatorial regions still live naturalistically as part of their respective ecosystems. The metabolic demand to maintain body heat encountered in arctic environments and the need to dissipate heat in tropical environments is the result of a basic character of geography and ecology.

There is therefore a geographic dimension to the nutritional needs of people. This, of course, is modified by the introduction of cultural factors, which alter patterns of activity or living as well as the environment itself. For example, Europeans entering into a tropical environment generally eat more than the indigenous people, because their activity patterns are markedly stepped up in comparison to the natural activity patterns of the indigenous populace.

Environmentally Induced Patterns of Nutrition

The EPC model suggests a search for cultural patterns of nutrition which are set by environmental or geographical factors.

A polarity can be discerned from a ruderal comparison of arctic peoples with tropical peoples. There are a number of human cultures among arctic populations, all of whom are herders or hunters. Some fishing enters into their largely subsistence economy, but the mainstay of life among them is the flesh of mammals. Eskimos are the familiar example to us, but on the Eurasian continent other groups such as the Laplanders, Tungus and Chuckchi live by similar modes of life in similar environs.

On the other hand, populations of tropical regions, whether of plains, savanas or mountains, are largely vegetarian in dietary habit. From time to time we read of the protein shortage among African people. This requires a closer look, there being an estimated 400,-000,000 cattle, goats and sheep on the continent, south of the Sahara alone. In addition there are now and have always been, contemporary with man, huge herds of bovid antelopes and other herbivores. Despite the value of these animals as "lobolla" or bride-price animals, the people of all herding and farming tribes kill and eat the flesh as desired. It is simply too basic for mankind not to eat flesh if the two conditions, availability and hunger, exist together. The tropical environment affords a sufficiency of plant food materials to at least sustain life, or we should not be hearing of vast population growth.

It has been described elsewhere that Eskimo diets are close to the physiologic tolerance of high protein and fat intake and of low intake of carbohydrates and Vitamin C. The principle plant group of arctic regions that affords any vegetable food at all for arctic populations is of the family Ericaceae, of which blueberries are most abundant. These are high in Vitamin C content, and in a way, may be viewed as a gift of nature to provide at least a minimal supply of this need.

Among tropical peoples, starchy foods are well-known. The ancient Quechua-Inca people of the Andean highlands are said to have cultivated more than a hundred kinds of potatoes. In Africa, millet is very common, used for "posho," a gruel-like cream of wheat, and also "pombe," a beer. There are many other starchy foods, such as rice, yams and cassava. Groundnuts are abundant and widely distributed throughout equatorial parts of Africa.

These environments, polar and equatorial, extreme in geographic or environmental differentiation, have certain natural productive attributes which meet the needs of human physiology, at least at minimal levels, or the regions could not have had a long, long history of human occupance. It would appear that a certain adequacy exists despite the knowledge generated by nutritional experimentation that leads us to a kind of crusade to change the dietary and other cultural habits of other peoples.

From personal experience, I can recall trips by dog team in the arctic when I melted "dog tallow" (beef tallow used for dog feed) and drank the drippings. The cold weather creates a craving for flesh and fat. It has been reported by Steffanson in journals of the American Medical Association that he lived healthfully under observation on a diet of meat and fat alone for a year. Body weight and vigor were maintained. In further personal experience in tropical Africa and South America, I found a keen desire for fruits and fleshy vegetables far out-weighing any craving for "red meat" and certainly felt no desire for fat such as one develops during arctic winters. Much of the meat consumed by Africans is first smoke-dried and precious little fat is found on any wild or domestic beast of those regions.

Turning to the temperate zone, lying between the polar and equatorial extreme, the land masses of Europe, Asia and America are notoriously rich in biological productivity. This diverse and bountiful productivity seems to have us in trouble. The Food and Nutrition Board of the National Research Council has announced a reduction of recommended dietary allowances from 2,900 to 2,800 calories per day for men, and from 2,100 to 2,000 calories per day for women. These recommendations, of course, are for people of average adult size, age and activity.

From these examples, a generalized version of a geographic pattern of environmental resistance, and activity to which nutritional needs are related, can be devised, shown as Figure 2.

LATITUDE	0 to 25	30 to 50	60 to 80
ENVIRONMENTAL RESISTANCE	LOW	MODERATE	HIGH
HUMAN ACTIVITY	RELATIVELY INACTIVE	MODERATELY ACTIVE	VERY ACTIVE

Fig. 2. Geographic pattern of environmental resistance.

To be fair about the matter, it probably should be considered that the activity patterns of populations in mid latitudes have been affected more by technology than have those of tropic and polar regions. The activity of "jogging," it would appear, is an effort to come to some balance between natural human physiology and modern human ecology, the latter impinging on physiology via technology, specifically mechanical labor aids.

Some Laws of Environment and Relationships to Human Ecology

Over the past century or two of scientific endeavor it would appear that much has been learned about plant and animal ecology and little of human ecology. However, much more is known than has been integrated into a formal "ecology of man" and those few books and papers bearing such titles have in general consisted of poorly related parts. The present paper, because of brevity, lacks depth, too.

On the other hand, animal ecologies and plant ecologies have been well composed, relating all the known life stages of plants and animals to the factors of environment known to impinge upon them. Not so with the ecology of man. The one outstanding block, it would appear, is the vastly accelerated pace of environmental change, artificialization of environment, and the great complexity resulting from culture. The components of this complexity, including smog and thermal pollution, may well prevent the formulation of any clear-cut human ecology on the same frame as wild plant or animal ecology.

If laws of environment exist they must be applicable to human populations as well as to plants and animals. Obscure as modern times make such an application, the idea of optimum environment, as conceived by the ecologist Shelford, provides an interesting analog.

Isolating one factor of environment, heat, an individual animal responds to heat as shown in Figure 3. Prairie dogs and ground squirrels are good examples of such a response to heat or cold, aestivating in summer and hibernating in winter. Extremes of temperature result in death.

HEAT FACTOR	VERY LOW	LOW	OPTIMUM RANGE	HIGH	VERY HIGH
RESPONSE OF INDIVIDUAL	DEATH	TORPOR (HIBERNATION)	ACTIVE	TORPOR (AESTIVATION)	DEATH

Fig. 3 Physiologic function of optimum environment.

Insofar as a population is composed of a number of individuals the population is responsive to the same environmental controls as the individual. It would therefore follow that population distribution should simulate such a pattern and the test model would appear as in Figure 4.

Return, now, to a map of world population to test this idea. The hottest of deserts and the polar ice caps should appear devoid, or nearly so, of human beings, and the densest of populations should be found in sub-tropical countries with mean monthly temperatures

ENVIRONMENTAL HEAT	VERY LOW	LOW	OPTIMUM	HIGH	VERY HIGH
POPULATION DENSITY	ABSENT	SPARSE	DENSE	SPARSE	ABSENT

Fig. 4. Hypothetic distribution of human population with respect to optimum environment.

approximating comfortable body temperature. The polar blanks labeled "uninhabited" agree well with the hypothesis. Tropical deserts which are labelled sparse or uninhabited also agree. Subtropical areas with more reasonable temperature regimes, from the stand-point of human body temperature, stand in fair agreement with this concept. The densely populated areas of Europe and North America do not agree, but these are areas where technical development has altered environmental conditions more drastically than elsewhere. A map of world population distribution illustrates some correlation of human population with a basic element of environment, heat.

Working from such a test and from the concept of the EPC model, certain laws or rules of environment that are known to pertain to plants and animals can be tested or examined in the context of a human ecology. One of these is a "First Approximation of Biotic Distribution."

Before a biotic distribution is possible a suitable environment for life is required. By observation and deduction life exists, therefore its environment is suitable; but not necessarily optimum. We next seek to explain the different forms of life found in different places. Eventually, it should be possible to describe the basic nature of human ecology, that is, on a naturalistic base. However, as time goes on and a greater and greater complexity develops from cultural and technological advances, it must be acknowledged that the whole context of ecology changes from a natural base to an artificial base. Perhaps the big question then becomes one of human evolution. Can the physiology of the human being change fast enough to match the pace of environmental change?

Considering the long evolutionary history of man and other mammals it would appear that man is destined to be earth-bound and had better learn to live within the framework of the natural environment in which we evolved. This sets the stage for examining the more natural and fundamental principles of human ecology, with less emphasis on the technical and higher cultural and social problems.

Many biologists have contemplated the origin of life. The processes of the corpuscularization and vitellization of life are known at least in outline and with due regard for brevity can be outlined as follows:

1. Life is a physico-chemical condition dependent upon heat (vant Hof's rule).

2. The origin of life occurred where heat was available for the physico-chemical process, in our frame of reference, in the tropics.

3. Conversely, ice caps and cold belts are devoid of life or poorly populated.

4. The heat belt of Earth was not always as it is now (see 9).

5. A shift of healt belts resulted in natural selection; fewer species survived adverse conditions than favorable ones. More species survived in the higher heat belt (see 8b). Also genetic varieties survived in amenable environments.

6. Revolutionary conditions of climate and physiography resulted in dissection of any belt-like distributions that might have existed, for example, as a result of continental drift.

7. Floras and faunas are reduced in number of species in progressively colder belts, to near sterility on ice caps (see 3).

8. The "simple" floras and faunas represent mutations "pre-adapted" to pioneering, and dispersed divergently from "hearth areas"; or are residual mutant populations (relicts; Sequoia-Redwood).

    a. The "advance" of simple floras and faunas follows glacial recession; glacial advance forces the recession of floras and faunas.

    b. Throughout geologic time permutations of mutations have repeated the pattern as a result of revolutionary climate and physiography.

    c. Therefore "disappearances" of some species have occurred but not necessaily "extinctions" (Hall 1946).

    d. Otherwise, we should have to invent a separate spontaneous generation of species for each epoch and for all places.

9. The shift of heat belts may have been shifts of radiation intensity rather than of geodesic position, that is, variations in solar radiation.

    a. or shifts in geodesic position with reference to the solar system

    b. or both

Then this results in latitudinal distributions obvious in extant species as well as in fossil forms, dependent upon the distribution of heat belts.

10. Vertical zonations, now existing, simulate in space the ontology of floras and faunas in time.

    a. Vertical zonations are accounted for by variations of radiation, lapse rate of temperature, precipitation regimes, and have changed with diastrophism, orogenesis, subsidence, pluvials, interpluvials, etc.

Laws or Rules of Environment

Laws and rules in the natural world are rarely really firm. That is to say, nature is so variable, the factors of environment are so changeable, as to make difficult the replication of conditions in order to test or prove laws of natural environment.

However, at this point I shall adopt the views of Mayr (1956), who defends some concepts which he calls "eco-geographical rules," but will use my own term "laws of environment" to illustrate some observed relationships of human adaptation to environment.

Mayr adopts the concept of a phenotype, that is any living thing, plant or animal, as representing a final compromise of innumerable selective pressures exerted by environment. The geographer recognizes innumerable variation of such factors of environment as temperature, humidity, pressure, altitude and so forth as representing regional variations on the earth's surface.

There is an extreme variation in the form of warm blooded animals but all have one thing in common, a rather constant body temperature of about 100° F (38° C). These are called homeotherms and include all races of man. Among the more obvious variations are the differences in fur or hair coats of mammals, and the clothing of men, of which environmentally induced variations are well known, ranging from gee string to burnoose among men, and naked skin to thick fur among wild mammals.

Less obvious are those variations of body bulk in relation to skin surface area. A German naturalist, Carl Bergmann, tested this idea in 1848, and found a geographical variation in the ratio of body volume to body surface area, within a given taxon, best illustrated at the generic level. For example among the hares, the heavier hares are found in northern regions, and the lighter in southern regions. Although a jackrabbit looks very large, it is actually much lighter than an arctic hare and has a higher ratio of surface area to body volume than the arctic hare. This is the basis of Bergmann's Rule and is regarded as a heat conservation adaptation.

Allen observed a similar phenomenon in the appendages of mammals and birds. Using the same example, hares, the ears of the arctic hare are very short while those of the jackrabbit are very long. These differences in the surface areas of the ears of these two closely related animals are believed to be phenotypic adaptations to environment, the former to *reduce* heat loss, the latter to *induce* or increase heat loss.

An application of these ideas to the ecology of man has been made by the anthropologists Howells (1960), Newman (1953), and others. In all fairness, it must be admitted that some anthropologists object to this analogy and even object to the original hypothesis pertaining strictly to animals other than man (Scholander 1955). The illustration, borrowed from Howells, shows these principles as applied to human ecology (Figure 5).*

Geographic Dimensions of Productivity

Biological productivity patterns respond to climatic controls and can also be described as a food crop geography. The underlying element of control is temperature and specifically the cardinal temperatures, those temperatures which are critical for the growth of various kinds of food crops. For each species of food crop there

---

*Reprinted from Distribution of Man by William W. Howells. Copyright 1960 by *Scientific American, Inc.* All rights reserved.

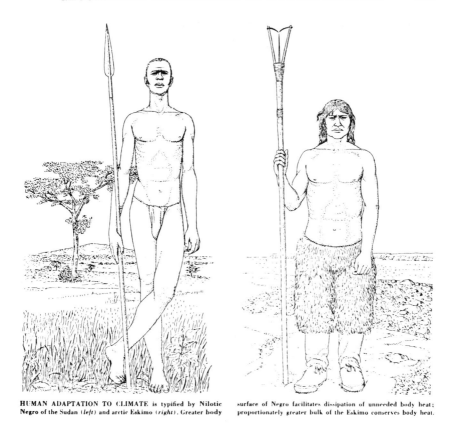

HUMAN ADAPTATION TO CLIMATE is typified by Nilotic   surface of Negro facilitates dissipation of unneeded body heat;
Negro of the Sudan (*left*) and arctic Eskimo (*right*). Greater body   proportionately greater bulk of the Eskimo conserves body heat.

Fig. 5. Application of laws or rules of environment to human physiology.

are maximum, minimum and optimum temperatures for growth, in agreement with the principle of temperature control of growth as stated in vant Hof's rule.

Space permits only a few examples of cardinal temperature controls which result in a geographic distribution of particular food crops. Oats, rye, wheat and barley, very closely related grains, have about the same temperature ranges, and the world distribution pattern of these grains are quite similar. Sorghum, maize and mellons have similar requirements, but the cardinal temperature range is higher than for the grains noted above. Therefore, the distribution of these food crops is somewhat more southerly than the hard grains. Differential crop distributions and related cultural patterns lead to a search for the origins of domestic food crop production.

Origins of the Acculturation of Environment
For the Improvement of Human Nutrition Supply

A knowledge of the origins of domestic crops and herds is likely to provide some explanation of present distributions and resultant cultural patterns. This subject is one of great intrigue, and great debate. Many scientists and philosophers have sought answers to the question of the origin of domestic plants and animals but because origins are tied up with evolution no one will ever know the whole story.

The plant ecologist, Holdridge (1967), has provided a concept based on purely environmental factors and tested in the real world of natural plant communities. Holdridge's theory is well based on physico-chemical laws using the most fundamental of environmental characteristics, temperature and precipitation. The inter-play of these elements of environment and organic physiologic processes in the form of respiration and transpiration result in the phenomenon of evapotranspiration.

Holdridge has perceived the balance of these phenomena to result in a "unity line," that is, a balance of precipitation, temperature and biotic processes in a ratio of one to one, or "unity." By a direct application of this idea to geographic place, Holdridge found that 19 of 21 major cities in South America had climatic characteristics of the "unity line." He inferred from this that the locations of these cities were very, very ancient, and represented geographic positions where the gaining of a livelihood was easiest. It therefore offered an optimum habitat for primitive people to experiment with the cultivation of wild food crops and the herding of wild ungulates. From an ecological point of view this environment also offered a variety of plants and animals with which to experiment.

A summary of Holdridge's concept in relation to human ecology can be illustrated by a diagram on which the unity line is drawn (Figure 6). In arid regions, in order to form a permanent, primitive agriculture, some form of irrigation is required. In humid regions, there is a continual struggle to clear forests which impeded permanent primitive agriculture. Where the arid-humid characteristics were near balance, the environment was more amenable to the development of permanent primitive settlement. This is offered by Holdridge

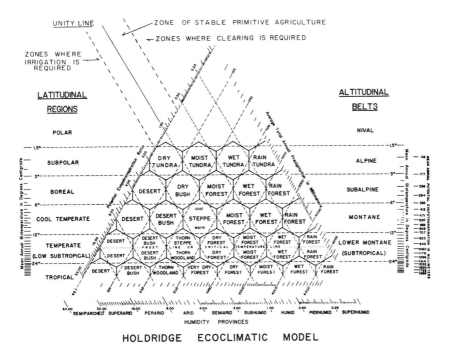

Fig. 6. Ecological basis for the development of a primitive, stable agriculture.

as an explanation of the location of most of the large cities of South America, and by extrapolation, some clue to the basic character of human ecology.

World Patterns of Food Production

Any good atlas reveals a generalized pattern of food crop production. This pattern, really composed of many patterns, has an obvious geographic quality. There are boundaries marking geographic differentiations.

For example, the pattern of coffee production is strictly tropical. The production of rye is practically confined to north temperate regions, none being produced in the Southern Hemisphere. Wheat is almost entirely extra-tropical in distribution and, as the main ingredient of bread, its use is well confined to those regions, *despite* a thoroughly developed transportation and economic exchange system. In other words, there is a strong geographic correlation of envionmental and cultural characteristics of specific geographic regions. Rice, yams and cassava (Manihot) are more examples of food production patterns, generated by environmental conditions, and leading to cultural patterns of food consumption.

The geography of intoxicating beverages is a cultural study in itself. It would seem that all the families of man have discovered the fermentation process and the effects of imbibition of the product. To illustrate the geographical nature of beverage production, the numerous wines of various regions of Spain, France, Portugal and ohter countries carry famed place names like Sherry, Burgundy and Port.

In Africa, a beer, "pombe," is made of millet, while the same kind of liquor is made in northern latitudes of malted barley, not found at all in Africa. There is, then, some pattern in the cultural fabric, related to environment, even in regions with higher levels of technology.

The Ecology of Malnutrition

The title of this section of this paper is taken directly from a group of six volumes in a Medical Geography Series compiled by Jaques May, M.D. (1950—).

In a perusal of these volumes, I have not found them to live up to their title. But this is not to negate the value of May's work. On the other hand, it has stimulated some thinking and constitutes a recording of food production in many parts of the world as well as some estimate of the patterns of food consumption in both developed and under-developed countries. The matter of the geography of malnutrition is only vaguely documented and one is left wondering if it exists at all.

One may find in the Statesman's Yearbook (1967-68), production, export and import records of food stuffs for most countries of the world. It is astonishing, in the light of popular notion, to find that many countries on the list of undernourished peoples are exporters of large quantities of food materials. India, for example, is reported to have exported tea, sugar, hemp, sisal, rice and wheat in 1968.

In at least some so-called underdeveloped countries of the world, surpluses of food are produced, and this has the effect of keeping thes countries at the agrarian level, unable to achieve the demographic transition which is characteristic of the Western World of the 20th Century. Uganda, Kenya, Colombia and Peru are examples.

Deshler's report (1963) on cattle in Africa provokes inspection of this situation. In 1959, 104 million cattle were reported in 50 territories of Africa south of Sahara. From the experience of all who have attempted such censuses, we know these to be underestimates and Deshler reports that veterinary departments consider these estimates to be as much as 20 percent below actual cattle populations.

In addition to cattle, there are millions of goats and sheep in Africa. Tauber, in an unpublished thesis (1967), has made a detailed study of goat and sheep production in northern Nigeria. These animals provide hides and skins valuable on the world leather market but of no use in Nigeria. The production of thousands of hides for this relatively small geographic area means the availability of thousands of pounds of meat. It is all consumed. None is wasted.

Tauber has devised a "geocthnograph" (Figure 7) to illustrate the relationship of geographic and cultural factors among several groups of people in northern Nigeria. By extension, this diagram shows the pattern of basic human ecology at the nomadic herding level of economic development.

Although these are but a few examples drawn from such sources as the Statesman's Yearbook, world atlases and published reports, the vast bulk of information really leads us to the conclusion that the world is producing an appalling amount of food and that much of this productivity is governed by the basic environmental factors in distinct geographic patterns. Superimposed over this productivity pattern, some cultural characteristics with respect to food habits and customs are generated. To some considerable extent, human physiologic needs are induced by environmental factors. At lower levels of economic or technologic development the characteristics of human ecology are naturalistic. At advanced levels the characteristics are artificial.

The Geography of Disease

The ecology of man must necessarily include diseases and debilitations which affect human populations. There are well known diseases with distinct geographic distributions. Malaria is one of these.

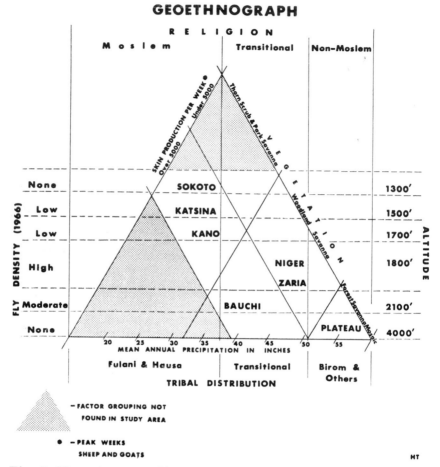

Fig. 7. Illustrating geographic and ecologic relationships which constitute the basic framework of human ecology in a semi-nomadic herding economy.

Morbidity in a population is to some extent a nutritional problem although there are many diseases which cannot be combatted by dietetic methods at all.

Probably all morbid conditions, whether nutritional or pathogenic, are part of an ecologic system. Indeed, many disease control methods are based on a knowledge of life cycles and utilize the principle of striking at the most vulnerable stage.

Some evidence leads to the conclusion that malnutrition and disease are cause and effect. Certainly, the maintenance of vigor through proper nutrition is some safeguard against disease, but a purely etiologic analysis of most diseases indicates only a low correlation of disease incidence with malnutrition. On the other hand, there are good correlations of geographical-ecological characteristics with the distribution of disease. The fundamental patterns are the same as those of other biotic distributions and based upon the laws of environment and physico-chemical rules such as vant Hof's rule as cited previously in this paper.

The generalized geographic pattern of biotic distribution includes diseases and parasites, there being a complexity of species in the heat belt regions and a paucity of species in polar or frigid regions. There is much more to this subject than can be treated within the scope of this paper, and a somewhat more detailed presentation can be found in the Yearbook of Agriculture, Climate and Man (1941).

By no means is this all there is to human ecology but this is much of the basic frame of the human relationship to environment. The technological age has generated ecological problems far more deleterious and foreboding for mankind than food shortage, but this time and this place are not appropriate for the long and complicated consideration necessary to describe or define all of the geographic dimensions of human ecology.

REFERENCES

Allee, W. C., O. Park, A. E. Emerson, T. Park and K. P. Schmidt, 1949. *Principles of Animal Ecology,* W. B. Saunders, Philadelphia, Pa.

Bresler, J. B., 1966. *Human Ecology,* Addison-Wesley, Reading, Mass.

Deevey, Edward S., 1960. The Human Population. *Scientific American,* September.

Deshler, Walter, 1963. Cattle in Africa. *The Geographical Review,* Vol. LIII, No. 1.

Hall, E. Raymond, 1946. *Mammals of Nevada.* University of California Press.

Holdridge, L. R., 1967. *Life Zone Ecology.* Tropical Science Center, San Jose, Costa Rica.

Howells, William W., 1960. The Distribution of Man. *Scientific American,* September.

May, Jaques, 1950 etc. in six volumes, *The Ecology of Malnutrition.* Medical Geography Series, U.S. Army, Natick Laboratory.

Mayr, Ernst, 1956. Geographic Character Gradients and Climatic Adaptation. *Evolution,* Vol. 10, No. 3, pp. 15-26.

Newman, Marshall T., 1953. The Application of Ecological Rules to the Racial Anthropology of the Aboriginal World. *American Anthropologist,* Vol. 55, No. 3, pp. 311-327.

Scholander, P. F., 1955. Evolution of Climatic Adaptation in Homeotherms. *Evolution,* Vol. 9, No. 1, pp. 15-26.

Statesman's Yearbook, Sternberg, S. H., ed. 1967-68. St. Martin's Press.

Tauber, Henry E., 1967. A Geographic Study of the Goat and Sheep Skin Industry of Northwest Nigeria. Unpublished master's thesis, University of Colorado.

World Atlas, 12th Edition, 1964. Rand McNally.

Yearbook of Agriculture, Climate & Man. 1941. U.S. Dept. of Agriculture.

SOME CROSS-CULTURAL UNIVERSAL AND NON-UNIVERSAL FUNCTIONS, BELIEFS, AND PRACTICES OF FOOD

MADELEINE LEININGER, Ph.D., R.N.
Dean, School of Nursing
University of Washington
Seattle, Washington

Probably no topic has universally intrigued man more than food. It is a subject which prehistoric man must have talked about considerably in his daily search for food in order to survive. Today, man seldom permits the topic of food to rest as he discusses food in his work and leisure time. Professional health personnel frequently talk about food in their efforts to modify man's eating practices in order to optimize man's use of food nutrients, to reduce body stresses or pathological states, and to prevent nutritional deficiencies. Both social and natural scientists are more and more involved and interested in the subject of food, studying man's food practices and beliefs in differing cultures and in the scientific study of the essential food elements for man.

Although food has long held scientific and humanistic interests, still there are a number of critical and important scientific questions which have not been answered to fully understand man's food behavior cross-culturally such as: 1) What universal criteria could be used to assess man's basic nutritional needs cross-culturally? 2) What are the basic nutritional needs of people in different cultures? 3) What is man's nutritional adaptation capacity under various ecological, cultural, social and psychological situations? 4) Where nutritional deficiencies exist in cultural areas, what universal or particularistic factors would account for their existence? 5) How is man's biological development affected by the availability and non-availability of food nutrients in various cultures? These questions and others await the collaborative research work of social scientists, nutritionists, physical scientists, ecologists, health scientists, and others interested in pursuing answers to these questions.

The central purpose, however, of this paper is to identify some of the universal and non-universal functions, beliefs, and practices of food cross-culturally with the intent of providing a broad framework of understanding man's food behavior and to assist helping agents to use this knowledge as they work with people having different cultural backgrounds. Examples from Western and non-Western cultures will be used to highlight the statements or postulates under discussion. In the first part of the paper some universal features and functions of food will be discussed, followed by a presentation of some non-universal aspects of food.

If one knew the food patterns of people in a particular culture, one would have a fairly reliable picture of man's current and past behavioral tendencies, his social interests, his evolutionary development, his biological makeup, and his cultural life patterns. In fact, cultures communicate *what they are* and *what they do* through the use of food. Food, then, is the important medium to understand and predict people's behavior. Let us turn to further ideas about the universal and non-universal functions, beliefs, and practices of food.

First, food is used universally to provide body energy and to satisfy man's biophysiological hunger. That man needs food for survival is well documented throughout the history of man. The human body is dependent upon a variety of food nutrients for its functioning and maintenance. Unquestionably, there are certain basic food nutrients which man must have for basic functioning and to exist. To date there are no ethno-scientific studies to document these basic nutritional elements cross-culturally. Ethnographic data suggests, however, that man tends to require different amounts of nutrient elements being dependent upon man's biological and hereditary makeup, his daily energy expenditure, his metabolic tendencies, his sociocultural life style, and other factors. We, too, know that if man does not receive minimal food nutrients (largely defined by his culture), one can anticipate nutritional deficiencies, sociocultural limitations, and other untoward consequences. Death, too, can be a consequence of man receiving limited foods for his biophysiological needs. A point of interest can be noted here. Although food is imperative for human energy and survival, some men do not always perceive the intake of food for this primary reason. Instead, man may deny his biological needs for food and use sundry reasons for consuming food. Nevertheless, food is still necessary for man's biological needs and to assure his survival.

Second, food is used universally to initiate and maintain interpersonal relationships with friends, kinsmen, strangers. As we know from our own American culture, food is an important means to initiate contacts with strangers and to maintain relationships with people. Through time, food has become the symbolic medium to achieve interpersonal relationships with people. Concomitantly, food serves as a definite organizing force to bring individuals and groups together and to keep them in contact with one another for varying periods of time. Food promotes individual relatedness with other beings — humans and non-humans. It is extremely important in developing group relationships, promoting social interests, and stimulating social cohesion. Probably no other object or substance is so important as food in fostering social relationships and in maintaining contacts with others. To illustrate this point, the use of the American coffee break will be discussed below.

Coffee and the coffee break has become a significant cultural item and practice in our society. Coffee (or its substitute) has become the symbolic means by which people get to know one another, to test social relationships, and to learn about another individual or group of people. The coffee break has developed as an institutional practice with a variety of interesting ritualized activities and functions — all of which center upon having a cup of coffee with other persons. The coffee break has not only become an important way to initiate new social contacts, but it is also an important means to explore social and occupational interests of people.

Several psychosocial and cultural functions of the coffee break have emerged in our culture. The coffee break provides an opportunity: 1) to meet new people; 2) to express emotional frustrations and tensions; 3) to gossip about and with others; 4) to boast about one's social and occupational achievements; 5) to explore personal and work problems with others; 6) to enhance feelings of self-esteem and identity; 7) to nurture group cohesion and social belongingness; 8) to communicate common or dissimilar life experiences; and 9) to work toward the solution of personal life problems.

One can see from these functions the important and diverse purposes of the coffee break. Indeed, the original intent of the coffee break, which was to serve as a short recess from one's routine work, has far exceeded it's initial purposes and expectations. In most institutions, coffee breaks have become one of the most important and "looked for" informal experiences in the work day of the employee. Job satisfaction, morale, and opportunities for new social ties (or the reaffirming of old ones) are largely contingent upon the coffee break and its multi-purposes. Of course, "tea breaks," "coke breaks," and "cocktail breaks," and other "liquid breaks" are other substitutes for the well known coffee breaks and the functions of these other "liquid breaks" are similar to that of the coffee break.

The use of food for communication and social relatedness is known in the history of *Homo sapiens* with many ways to show that food has both social and communication purposes. The processes, however, in the use of food vary with different cultural groups as to how food is used for socio-communication purposes. There are, however, some recurrent expectations and patterns of behavior which one can identify between the food-giver and food-receiver which has cross-cultural relevance.

To begin with, usually, there are culturally defined game rules to achieve some relative degree of equality in the process of giving and receiving of food over a period of time. The norms of the culture will usually determine the social (or etiquette) rules as well as the ritualized practices related to food giving and receiving. Safe social chit-chat, the recognition of persons giving the food, and the overt acknowledgement of the status or position of the food-giver are generally part of the initial giving of food. Usually, this behavior is followed by more formalized rules of serving, distributing, or presenting food to specified persons. It is always important to formally recognize people who have attained a defined social position if he is the food-giver as it "adds to" his social status.

Then, as the receiver(s) are given the food, they must acknowledge (in their culturally defined ways) their feelings of gratefulness and appreciation for the food. The time, place, size of the group, participants, and the cultural context are all important variables in fostering social communication and relatedness to others in food giving and receiving activities. In the process of giving and receiving of food, one can observe not only the formal and informal patterns of behavior, but also the amount and kind of communication and interaction which occurs. Social relatedness may be significantly increased or decreased during the course of any food giving and receiving, and it is well to note what does actually occur in such food exchanges.

Closely related to the above function of food, is the *third function, namely to determine the nature and extent of interpersonal distance between people.* Perhaps this statement can best be understood by the author's own personal experiences with a group of people from the Eastern Highlands of New Guinea. The author lived with two Gadsup village groups for approximately thirteen months, spending seven and six months with each village group. During this time, she systematically observed and recorded the quantity and quality of food given to her as a stranger by the native people during the course of her stay with the peoples.

It was, indeed, interesting to discover that during the first two weeks in both villages, only small amounts of withered, scrubby, and less desirable foods were offered to the ethnographer. The people cautiously offered the food to her and were intensely interested in observing her actions and general behavior. The behavior of the Gadsups was a direct reflection of their attitudes and responses to a white, strange and unknown female. For it was true that initially, the people were very cautious, frightened, and inquisitive of the female ethnographer. Actually, they feared her as a potential sorceress in their village.

Toward the end of the second week, the amount of food increased slightly, but the quality of food had not changed from what was offered during the first two weeks. At this time, the people were beginning to feel a bit more comfortable with the ethnographer; however, they were uncertain of her actions, role, and interest in them. By the end of the fourth week, the villagers were considerably more relaxed with the ethnographer, and consequently, the quality of the food improved noticeably and the amount of food offered to the researcher increased. And towards the end of her stay in the villages, the ethnographer was besieged with choice and special foods, many of which the people walked a great distance to obtain.

Thus food became an important means to determine interpersonal distance and social relatedness with a group of non-Western peoples. It was also interesting to note that the more acculturated Gadsup villagers used food as a vehicle to relate to the ethnographer more extensively than did the less acculturated village group. The latter group was not so adept in using food for social relatedness with Western people, but rather used their own natural, personal, and cultural ways to relate to a stranger.

A fourth universal function of food is for the expression of socio-religious ideas. Cross-culturally, food is used importantly and dis-criminately for a variety of socio-religious activities in order to com-municate certain cultural messages and for multiple symbolic pur-poses. The quality and quantity of food varies when used for ceremonial religious and social activities. In addition, the number of people involved in preparing and serving the foods varies with different cultures and according to the specific ceremony being conducted. Usually, the choice of food and the amount is a clue to the significance and status of the ceremony. For example, in many cross-cultural religious ceremonies which honor the dead or their ancestors, only choice foods and large amounts of food are used in the ceremony and this is a sign of great honor, respect, and reverence for the dead.

Displays of food at harvest ceremonies are another common prac-tice in many places in the world in order to celebrate the abundance of food produced and the gratefulness of the people to supernatural and natural forces for making the food possible. Generally these ceremonies are colorful, happy, and religious occasions. The people usually wear bright festive costumes at these harvest ceremonies. Gratefulness for the foods is shown by the people praying, singing, and performing special ritual acts of appreciation. The ceremony is a public affair with many local people participating actively in the festivities.

Birth ceremonies are another example in which foods are used in special ways to symbolize a child's entry into the community and to express the wishes and desires of the people for the child who will soon be socialized as a full participating adult member of the community. For instance, during the Gadsup birth ceremony, the uncle of a two-month old infant is given small particles of native food to taste. These foods are ones which the Gadsup people have raised in their gardens. As the father's brother places the food on the infant's tongue, he says these words: "We give you these foods from our gardens so that you will want these foods and will work hard to grow them." This beautiful and simple birth ceremony used food as the primary symbolic way to convey the villagers hope that the infant will grow strong, have a great desire to raise Gadsup foods, and be a true Gadsup adult.

In our United States culture, one can note how the kinds and amounts of food vary with two festive socio-religious ceremonies, namely, Thanksgiving and Christmas. Traditionally, certain foods have been selected as preferred foods for each occasion. For instance, turkey, dressing, sweet potatoes, and cranberries have long been selected as preferred foods for Thanksgiving Day; whereas, a variety of roasted meats, plum pudding, Christmas cookies, candy, and other special delicacies are foods selected for Christmas Day. Generally, a large amount of food is accumulated and prepared for these two festive days—much more than one usually finds daily in the home.

In most cultures, foods used at ceremonial feasts not only vary in quantity and quality, but the foods are usually expensive, exotic, scarce, highly preferred, and require special cooking and serving. These features make the foods even more special and make the ceremony a never-to-be-forgotten day. Still another closely related feature of socio-religious ceremonial activities is that before a large ceremony there is usually the practice of food taboos. The recognition of food taboos associated with ceremonies has been known for many years with many culture groups. Abstinence from eating tabooed foods (which are generally choice and desired foods) makes the people who have observed the food taboo very desirous of the special foods. The tabooed food increases in value, status, and importance. Tabooed foods are usually given to the people at the end of the ceremony or at a specified time in the future.

A fifth universal function of food is the use of food for social status, social prestige, and for special individual and group achievements. To publicly acknowledge that an individual has achieved or been ascribed to a certain social status is an impressive occasion. However, the use of specifically prepared foods to validate the fact gives the individual and group added recognition and social prestige. Expensive and choice gourmet foods are often used to communicate that an individual or group has changed status and role in the community.

One of the best examples to highlight how an individual or group gains public recognition is the male initiation rites which are practiced in many places in the world. Initiation rites are a colorful and impressive ceremony, but usually harsh for the new initiates. Initiation rites are highy symbolic ceremonies to symbolize that an individual has moved from one social position to another in a given community, e.g., from a boy to a man.

Prior to the initiation ceremony, the initiates are expected to observe strict food taboos and to bravely accept the ritualized acts administered to them. At the end of the ceremony and after they have performed a number of rigorous activities to test their manliness, they are given the tabooed foods. Every culture selects what their tabooed foods will be and what rules they will use in giving the food to them. Many of the rituals, beliefs, and practices associated with initiation rites have continued for many generations with limited food elaborations and changes. In general, the initiation ceremony remains a highly symbolic one with the use of special foods as the means for helping the initiates realize that they have achieved a desired social position and status in the community.

Although we do not have such definitive initiation rites in our culture, still there are ways that we give public recognition to the adolescent. Most noticeably is when an adolescent has reached twenty-one years of age, has acquired a driver's license, or has achieved some special recognition. His parents and close nuclear kinsmen help him celebrate the occasion by preparing special foods he likes, honoring him at a social gathering, and permitting him some "extra" social privileges. The movement of the adolescent into his new social status tends to vary in our culture with the socio-economic class of his parents. Our culture is also accustomed to using food to show a change in one's mode of living as a person moves from a lower class to an upper social class. Again, gourmet or special foods are often used to communicate such changes in status.

A sixth universal function of food is to help cope with man's psychological stresses and needs. More and more foods are being used to allay man's internal and external tensions, and quite apart from their ability to satisfy man's hunger needs. The gorging of food and the compulsive eating of food and drinks (and usually limited cognitive awareness of what is happening to an individual) are frequently signs of psychological tension. Individuals, too, hoard large amounts of food without realizing their appropriate usage. Such behavior becomes most apparent to mental health personnel as they work with clients who are under emotional stress. Food has become an important way people have learned to deal with emotional tensions and crisis situations. Compulsive eating of food to allay tension tends to increase with the perceived or actually felt tensions of the individual.

Occasionally, an individual under great stress will not eat food. These persons are generally quite depressed and unable to mobilize enough energy to get food, or more importantly, they do not feel they are worthy to receive foods. This pattern of using food to handle stress is most apparent with people in the United States culture where food plays such a large part in our lives and is easily available to most people, except for poverty groups. Cross-culturally, food is used to deal with threats, overt crisis, and anxiety-producing situations.

As a side interest, the author has often asked undergraduate students what food they used most frequently to cope with emotional and social stresses, and their reply was "milk." Milk in many ways symbolizes the comfort, contentment, and security of life as it was at home in the early days. When graduate students were asked this same question, their most frequent response was a "drink and an up-tight pill." Graduate students tend to resort to soft and hard drinks and to medications to quickly suppress their anxiety or to provide a special extrasensory experience. Their goal is to make themselves become less "tight" and to increase their social interaction with colleagues, or to have a special psychological happening with

hallucinogenic subtsances. Some graduate students said that hard
liquor or tranquilizing pills helped them to control themselves through
a crisis and to "get the most out of life." Thus food and drink
serve as crucial means to provide personal security, to bolster one's
self-esteem, to help express anger or frustration, to release oneself
from a world of tension, and to recapture earlier comfort and contentment kinds of experiences.

Closely akin, we find that food also supports man's attempt to
achieve self-actualization and self-gratification. But most importantly,
food is the means to cope with anxiety and frustrating life situations
which arise suddenly or maintain themselves over a period of time.
Food allays many internal stresses and provides energy to cope with
solutions to problems. Food is also used to relieve feelings of boredom
and prolonged dissatisfaction with life. Sweets and drinks are commonly used in our United States culture to cope with boredom and
to reward and comfort oneself. Sometimes, the consumption of
sweets suddenly affects one's physiological appearance without the
individual fully realizing what has caused the change in his body
appearance. Snacking and drinking not only reduces boredom in
our society, but also provides ways to increase interpersonal acceptance and social interaction.

*A seventh function of food is to reward, punish, or influence the
behavior of others.* Cross-culturally, people know the ways they wish
to influence adults and children in either a positive or negative
manner. In most cultures, positive and negative sanctions are ways
of getting tasks done and are a socializing means to make individuals
acceptable and functioning members of their society. Usually, sweets,
rare foods, or specially procured foods are used to reward an individual; whereas, unwanted or less preferred foods are used to punish
an individual. Sometimes, horribly distasteful foods are given to
individuals for punishment, such as hot peppers and slimy raw foods.
The particular foods used and their symbolic meaning for rewards
and punishment vary with different cultures.

Children in our culture learn very early the multiple ways to
influence adults by aversive or socially non-desirable behavior or
through the use of foods. They test parents to see what kind of
food behavior will be rewarded or punished, and at the same time

they are adept to highlight the ambiguities and inconsistencies of parents through the use of foods. A small child can generally elicit a good reaction from his parents by not eating food, being a highly picayunish eater, or by being a messy eater, particularly in front of the parents' friends. The adolescent, too, is capable in our society of communicating hostility, rebellion, and deviant behavior by the use of food. In sum, foods have been important means in our culture to socialize children and to reward, punish, and to influence adult and child behavior.

An eighth function of food is to influence the political and economic status of a group. Early man was quick to discover that food had good economic and political values. Politically, food has been used cross-culturally to build alliances with new groups of people, to reaffirm traditional and new political ties, and to test relationships of influence and power with others. Food is a powerful force to solidify precarious or tenuous relationships with different political groups. Serving food before, during, and after political meetings often dispels the "heat" and interpersonal tension found in arriving at major political decisions.

Cross-culturally, food is generally served to political participants as a symbol of political hospitality and to express basic trust and friendliness towards other men. Sometimes, food gifts are exchanged between political groups before or after the meetings. In some cultures, political leaders are most adept in offering potentially hostile or quarrelsome leaders some choice foods or drinks before the meeting to soften their aggressive or polemic dispositions. But most importantly, food is tremendous in building and extending political alliances with new and old political groups.

For example, the Gadsup people usually offer food to their political associates at gatherings in which both their traditional friends and enemies are present. They formally offer some choice foods to their traditional enemies and offer regular foods to their friends. The choice foods offered to their traditional enemies (and especially to men with noted political power) is done to reduce the threat of sorcery and to impress the "big men" of their brotherliness and generosity. Foods which are dried or not of prime status in appearance or consistency are always suspect, and enemies anticipate sorcery practices of the group.

Economically, food is important in exchange to maintain a basic food supply and in providing diversity in the people's diets. Since the economics of food is concerned with production, accumulation, and distribution, man learns how to influence his own status and others by these economic aspects. He imports or exports foods according to the needs, economic interests, and past trade relationship patterns with different cultures. Generally, food exchanges tend to increase the economic and social status of a group and also enhance the potential for new social ties with other groups. The whole topic of food economics is quite complex and extensive, and is beyond the scope of this paper. It is, however, important to keep in mind that the way people produce, distribute, and accumulate food is necessary to understand their food usage. It is also important to understand how the people have survived ecoonmically through time and how they continue to survive today in any culture.

Finally, but certainly not exhaustively, *food is used to detect, treat, and prevent social, physical and cultural behavior deviations and illness manifestations.* Food is often used as the first means to diagnose and treat an illness. In most cultures, a diagnostician or deviner uses food to detect socio-cultural and physical difficulties. Food is used to explain why certain illnesses occurred and to predict their possible consequences. Food is a medium for understanding a variety of factors which initiate, aggravate, or precipitate social tensions and illnesses. If food is spoiled or not of the right consistency, it is always possible that the giver(s) had malevolent or questionable intentions, and so one must explore past social relations and behaviors. In devination practices, food is used to warn people of potential threats from outsiders and to an entire social group.

Professional and non-professional people use foods in many ways to relieve symptoms of psychophysiological or social stresses and as a definite form of care and treatment. Cross-culturally, many of these forms of treatment and care with foods have not been studied systematically. Folk and scientific approaches to help sick people include ways to use food substances for specific and general treatment. Thus food is crucial in the prevention of illness and in the curative and remedial treatment of illnesses.

In the next section, some non-universal functions, beliefs, and practices will be identified with the view of highlighting factors influencing *differences* in food habits. Differences are important to understand why diversity in cultures exist and why changes in food practices may be difficult for some cultures as well as what facilitates rapid acceptance of new food practices.

Perhaps the most significant factor influencing differences in food practices is related *to the cultural values of a particular cultural group.* Cultural values are the sustaining life forces which determine the choices or preferences an individual or group make in their ways of living. They are the affective and cognitive tendencies that serve as powerful motivational forces to think and act in certain ways. Cultural values tend to be values which are not easily forgotten or highly subject to change. They serve as important guidelines for action and generally have a lasting and pervading influence on the people.

In our United States culture, many Americans place a high cultural value on meat, milk and milk products, fresh fruits, and some vegetables. In contrast, meat and milk products do not have a high cultural value as desired foods to consume in some parts of the world. For example, in India these foods are cultural taboos, as cows are viewed as sacred and cow's meat is not to be eaten. In other cultures, insects are choice foods; whereas, we reject them almost entirely. The Gadsup people of New Guinea give as their cognitively preferred foods: sweet potatoes, pork, and taro. When I offered them cake, bread, and candy, they politely tasted these foods. Later they told me that they disliked "my foods because they are mushy and have a strong taste." Thus the choice of foods and what foods will be eaten is largely determined, and one must not expect that another culture will readily accept our valued foods.

As a side interest, you may think by the choice of foods of the Gadsup people that they must be obese peoples. However, this is not true; there is no such thing as a fat Gadsup man, woman or child. The Gadsup people are of a muscular type, and are generally average for their age and height in body build. An obese Australian woman who weighed 250 pounds visited in one of my Gadsup villages. The Gadsup people were amazed at the size of the woman and consequently, I spent several days trying to explain to the Gadsups how the Australian woman could have become so large.

In the Mexican-American families which the author is now studying in an urban city area, the people gave as their first, second,
and third food preferences, tortillas, beans, and chile. These preferred foods exist for over approximately 52 percent of the families
and regardless of the fact that they have been living in a large
urban and highly acculturated community for more than sixteen
years. Other foods such as milk, meat, and fresh vegetables and
fruits, which other non-Mexican Americans are trying to make a
part of their diet, are of secondary value and are difficult to obtain
because of the low incomes of these families. From these examples,
one can see that cultural values in foods become a strong guiding
force in selection, production, and consumption of foods. Furthermore, agents of change must be aware of the people's food preferences
and use strategies to introduce food nutrients which are compatible
with the indigenous food values and beliefs.

Cultural beliefs and practices buttress and reinforce the indigenous
values of a particular group of people. However, these beliefs and
parctices vary with cultures and are non-universals. Beliefs in food
taboos and food usage are rooted in folk beliefs, cultural history,
religious beliefs, and sociocultural traditional practices, and so they
take on special meanings and forms of practice. Beliefs in animal
food taboos are commonly found in several cultures because animals
are often a symbol of an ancestral clan group. Therefore, the meat
from a totem animal is viewed as sacred and one which cannot be
consumed by the people of that culture.

Food taboos vary cross-culturally, and it is difficult to know these
taboos unless one has lived with or carefully studied the people.
Strangers may never know of them, but will wonder why people
do not eat certain foods they want them to eat. Food change agents
can be baffled by the people's resistance to new food practices if
they do not understand these food taboos. Animals, bird, and other
objects are used as tabooed and totem foods, and the practices and
beliefs related to food taboos are closely related to social structure
and organizational features of the culture. A host of other beliefs
and practices which are inextricably related to cultural values can
be identified in every culture. Some are highly particularistic and
non-universal.

Another important factor which influences differences in food practices is the environmental resources of the people. In some cultures, only certain kinds of food can be grown in the local environment. For example, in the Pacific Islands, the Micronesia people rely upon fish, breadfruit, and local nuts and fruits as their physical environment supports this kinds of food production. In India, rice, wheat, millet, and barley predominate, and milk products are limitedly available. The fauna and flora of an indigenous environment structures considerably what foods will be produced and nurtured generation after generation, and these foods usually became a part of the people's cultural values. Soil, climate, rainfall, and other factors found in an ecosystem also determine what foods will be or not be available to the people. This is particularly true in simple, non-technological societies where man and nature have developed a sensitive and intimate relationships with one another.

In our own highly developed nation, this intimate understanding between man and his environment is not so fully recognized. Commoner[1] states we are quite aware of the benefits of good technology, but we are also victims of it. He states:

"We are *unwitting* victims of environmental pollution, for most of the technological affronts to the environment were made, not out of greed, but ignorance. We produced automobiles that envelop our cities in smog — long before anyone understood its harmful effects on health. We synthesized and disseminated new insecticides — before anyone learned that they also kill birds and might be harmful to people. We produced synthetic detergents and put billions of pounds into our surface waters — before we realized that they would not be degraded in disposal systems and would pollute our water supplies. For a number of years we spread radioactive fallout across the globe — before we learned that the resulting biological risks made it too dangerous to continue. . . . Clearly, we have compiled a record of serious failures in recent technological encounters with the environment."

Thus the consequences of altering a complex natural ecosystem to produce different products felt more useful to a community can greatly influence the nutritional, health, and economic status of the people. In general, the evolution of the cultural patterns of people helps to stabilize the relation of man to his environment or to a particular ecosystem.

Closely related to the available environmental resources is the local economic pattern which influences differences in uses of food. An economy is concerned with the ways people make a living whether by horticulture, fishing, lumbering, industries, hunting, or sundry other means. It is concerned with the rationale, means, and cultural practices related to the production, consumption, and distribution of foods in a particular community. Through time, people not only chose their culturally preferred foods, but the economic pattern of producing and distributing the foods varies in most cultures. Economic factors such as male and female power to produce food are important; the method of distributing and producing foods; and the ultimate use of food, are all important variables related to food usage.

In most cultures, there are persons who assume economic roles and are quite knowledgeable about the people's weekly, monthly, and yearly consumption of food. Even though there are variations in the supply and demand of food, most economic leaders try to regulate a balance between the food use and food demands. In sum, multiple economic factors have to be considered in determining differences or non-universals of what foods will be used, consumed, distributed, rejected, and promoted by people in different communities.

Another fascinating factor which is just beginning to be recognized and understood as a definite influence on food usage is the *internal metabolic environment of man and its interaction with the external environment.* Essentially, the concern is with the flow of various nutrients, food and drink, from man's external environment to his internal environment with focus upon the utilization or non-utilization of nutrients. Genetic, constitutional, and metabolic processes of a particular cultural group differ and may be quite different from other cultural groups. Some human populations are intolerant of foods introduced by outsiders, and the foods may actually aggravate or threaten the health and survival of a culture. This fact has direct implications for people and agencies who contend that certain foods are extremely essential and must be given to a cultural group, and yet they may not realize that the people have a metabolic or genetic intolerance of the food. A few documented incidents have been reported by Bunce, Davis, and Bolin.

Dr. Bunce[2] reports a metabolic disturbance found in northeast Brazil in which the population was predisposed to any aggravation of Vitamin A deficiency. Dried milk was introduced into the community which caused the people to experience sudden growth. However, this led to a rapid depletion of the existing meager supply of Vitamin A. The consequences were an outbreak of night blindness, xerophthalmia, keratomalacia, and irreversible blindness. Thus Dr. Bunce offers a warning to people who have the good intention of improving dietary inputs in undernourished countries, as the foods may be highly disruptive to the normal metabolic functions of the people. Studies are certainly needed to evaluate and predict the consequences of introducing new foods into a culture.

Still another instance has been reported by Drs. Davis and Bolin[3] of Australia, who discovered that the absorption and digestion of milk is dependent upon the presence of the enzyme lactase. As we know, lactase is needed to break down lactose into two simple sugars, glucose and galactose. There is growing evidence that a number of people and other mammals in the world who produce the lactase enzyme in the intestine gradually cease to produce lactase after the infant stops ingesting the mother's milk. Consequently, when milk aid programs are introduced into different countries, complications ensue because of a primary lactase deficiency existing in the population. Following the ingestion of lactose, symptoms of diarrhea (often severe) and other related manifestations of a disturbed intestinal mucosa have been reported.

Cook and Kajubi[4] discovered an "inherited congenital" difference in lactase levels between different African tribes. In Baganda, lactase deficiency is common, occurring in 89 percent of the people. Their diet is primarily vegetable, consisting mainly of bananas. Davis and Bolin's study showed lactose intolerance to be common in Chinese students, New Guinea natives, and in a small group of Indians.

Although explicit data regarding the sampled population of these groups were not mentioned by the above researchers, still their findings serve as caveats for the introduction of milk and milk products into a culture without some knowledge of the community. At least the results give some indication of the communities that would benefit from the introduction of milk products and those that might have serious consequences of such a health program plan. If the lactose intolerance is an adaptive phenomenon, it is possible to introduce the milk gradually by increasing the lactose input from the various milk products. But if the lactose intolerance is genetically determined, then one would probably improve the nutrients in the cultural group's basic diet. These findings really make one aware of the need for more cross-cultural nutritional studies, and especially to understand metabolic processes, genetic tendencies, and their relationship to the environment of the people.

Although a number of other factors could be discussed which have a substantial influence on cultural differences in food use and practices, the author will only summarize these factors. Culture contact and acculturation processes can have a significant influence upon what foods a group of people may wish to adopt or to reject from another culture. When two or more cultures come in contact with one another, there are multiple factors which determine what a culture will or will not accept. One important factor is what the local people understand about the new foods which are being introduced into their food system. Generally, people try to conceptualize how the new foods will fit in with their current social, cultural, and food system, and if the foods seem congruent with their plan, they will probably accept them. If on the other hand, the foods are noncongruent, one can anticipate that they will be difficult to assimilate smoothly into their culture. Frequently, Western change agents like to use scientific data to help indigenous groups understand the rationale for changes. However, the "scientific facts" are usually different from the cognitive reference of the people, and so they may not be effective means to help people. Instead, facts used from the local people are often more effective and understandable to the indigenous peoples.

Food use, acceptance, and beliefs are also influenced by the way foods *relate to the beliefs in supernaturals, magic, sorcery, and curing*, and there are a great variety of beliefs and practices regarding these variables. Some food objects lend themselves more to supernatural and devination rites than others, and a cultural group is quick to recognize this point. Variability in food use will undoubtedly continue as magic, the supernatural, and sorcery continue to be practiced.

Social stratification is another factor producing differences in the way food is used. The way a society is stratified by castes, classes, and other methods determines who gets what foods and what foods will be used by the culture. In some stratified societies, certain foods are highly restricted to a particular class or caste, and it is culturally taboo to change this plan for social living. Furthermore, the foods are regulated by the caste and class, religious, social, political, and economic factors—all dependent upon this kind of food use and distribution.

Finally, food use *cross-culturally varies with the way food appears and is served to others*. Color, form, shape, consistency, and other factors do determine if an individual or group will select and eat the food. In some cultures, red may be a taboo color, and so any red foods may not be accepted. The way foods are prepared and served are non-universal features. Whether food is baked, boiled, grilled, fried, or prepared in multiple other ways determines the consumption and manner in which food is used. Accordingly, the way food is served determines the acceptance and enjoyment of foods.

In this paper, some cross-cultural universal and non-universal ideas about food have been presented. Hopefully, these ideas will help us to realize both the common and diverse features of food. The how, when, where, and what of food use and its functions are extremely important factors in understanding any cultural group. Since we are moving more and more toward a large world community of people, the challenge is even greater than one has conceived in the past to work and communicate effectively with many peoples in our world. Most important, we can use food as the medium to build trans-world relations, to promote optimal health for any cultural group, and to work toward the eradication of nutritional deficiencies. Now and for the future the reduction of food hunger will be our challenge and problem.

Before we can be an effective helper, however, we must use the knowledge which is available to us about world cultures. Anthropological knowledge is also valuable in dealing with people to facilitate rapid culture changes. Background knowledge about people gives a baseline for bringing about effective cultural changes. In addition, feelings of empathy and compassion for others can do much to facilitate our work efforts and good intentions of helping others. We need more creative thinkers, planners, and empathetic responders to work with people of other lands. New teaching methods and learning guidelines are also needed to understand and help others. The modes of learning and teaching others in non-Western societies are often quite different than found in our Western world. Thus, we urgently need new and creative teaching and learning approaches to help people in other countries.

Undoubtedly, as we become more involved in studying the food practices, beliefs, and functions of different cultures, we will discover the need for comparative research studies and approaches. We will realize how extremely important is knowledge of the way people live, in order to understand food use and beliefs. The "old fashions" of food use must be considered in the light of the "new fashions" of people. For how man has lived in the past, particularly in respect to food use, remains an interesting topic and one which can offer much "food for thought" in guiding changes for new food use and practices in the world.

REFERENCES CITED

1. Commoner, Barry. "Frail Reeds in a Harsh World," In *Natural History,* Vol. LXXVIII, No. 2, February, 1969, p. 44.

2. Bunce, G. Edwin. "Milk and Blindness in Brazil," In *Natural History,* Vol. LXXVIII, No. 2, February, 1969, pp. 52-53.

3. Davis, A. E. and T. D. Bolin "Milk Intolerance in Southeast Asia," In *Natural History,* Vol. LXVIII, No. 2, February, 1969, pp. 53-55.

4. Cook, G. C. and S. K. Kajubi. "Tribal Incidence of Lactase Defiicency in Uganda," *Lancet.* Vol. I, 1966, p. 725.

GENERAL REFERENCES

Jelliffe, B. Derrick. *Child Nutrition in Developing Countries.* Superintendent of Documents, U.S. Government Printing Office, Washington, D.C.

Lowenberg, Miriam E., E. Neige Todhunter, Eva D. Wilson, Moira C. Feeney, and Jane R. Savage. *Food and Man.* New York: John Wiley and Company, 1968.

Honigmann, John J. *Understanding Culture.* New York: Harper and Row, 1963.

Keesing, Felix. *Cultural Anthropology.* New York: Holt, Rinehart and Winston, 1965.

Leininger, Madeleine M. Gadsup Ethnography. Unpublished field notes, 1965.

DISCUSSION

QUESTIONS TO DR. QUICK AND DR. LEININGER

QUESTION: I work for Public Health, and I want to go on record that the Public Health Nutrition Programs are based on an in-depth history (most of them, I know) of what the family can afford, what they prefer, what they have, before anything else is told to them. The only changes made are those that are considered absolutely necessary. Our whole foundation in the Colorado area, our basis, is beans and tortillas. I would like to know just out of curiosity, who you are working with in the Denver Study and when your conclusions are going to be out, that kind of information.

ANSWER: (Dr. Leininger) I am working with 50 families in the so-called Goathill area. That is the section along the Platte River to the west of the river and the east of Federal Boulevard. In this section we selected really Spanish speaking families. We have both Mexican-American and Spanish-American in our sample. We have just completed the study of the 50 families, and we are now in the process of analyzing data. I hope within the next year I can get some of the results out on it.

It has been very interesting, although I regretted very much (and this is quite different from any anthropologist just coming in and spending time with them on Saturdays and Sundays, or during the week, too) that I really did not live right in the community. This is my only regret because I would have liked to live with them. We spent on an average at least seven to eight visits with each of the families, and I did have some people who participated because they were interested, graduate students in anthropology, some nurses who helped, and also Margaret Ball went out with me a couple of times, too. I think there is a wonderful opportunity to really get in and look at some of these things.

For instance, I think Margaret was surprised to find out the way they even canned food. They had canned a lot of their chile products in pop bottles, and I have seen them later during the last three years (I have been doing a longitudinal study), and very few have spoiled. They have kept them in the bottles, and this is their way of canning. Some families are very poor, and although I haven't finished the statistics on them yet, close to about 48 percent have income of less than $5,000 per year.

RESPONSE: (Dr. Theodoratus) I would like to make a comment myself, and that is that one particular dimension that I have become a bit more aware of in recent years, after becoming a parent, is the role of the peer group of small children in the problems of food and nutrition. Above all, this delightful one (which is perhaps not so delightful) that I am going through right now — the induction of a stress situation known as "fried liver." Not only one child or two children, but the entire group of about twenty other children in the next two blocks reinforce this particular attitude.

QUESTION: How much weight did you lose or did you maintain a lower weight when you were with these people, and how hot was it?

ANSWER: (Dr. Leininger) I lost fifteen pounds while I was over there, and I think most of it was when I went to the second village. The first was on a flat cunai area with just a little bit of bush in the extreme area, and the second village was on top of the mountain peak, about 400 to 500 feet. This is where I really lost it — in the climbing. I didn't know how to climb and I lost quite a bit there. But I felt good all the time I was there, and this was something I was a little concerned about — what happens if you get sick. At the beginning I had, I am sure, mostly traditional enemies. Who could I rely on? The closest town was about thirty or forty miles away, and of course, there is no modern communication system. The only way you could ever get in was to walk with the people or have them carry you in. So I was grateful that I stayed as healthy as I did, but I think, in terms of my nursing and medical background, that I had ways of protecting myself. I must say, for instance, when they offered me raw pork which is the way they eat it, I could never quite get that down.

I would usually take it into my little hut or in the outside shelter —
I had an open fireplace — and I would cook it well. Of course,
they don't have trichinosis and things like that, so some of these
organisms are not in that society.

Now with regard to the climate, during the wet season (they
have a wet and dry season) it does get quite cool. At night the
temperature goes down, during the wet season, to about 57
degrees. In the daytime it gets up to about 80 degrees. During
the dry season there is about a ten to twelve degree variation,
but the warmest it seemed to get was about 85 degrees. Yet we
were only six degrees from the equator, but it was a high mountainous area, as you could see, and a very pretty area, very colorful.
Everything grew there. I never saw anything like it; the snakes,
the bugs, *everything* grew. They were a huge size. I would see
something coming toward me, and I would think, "My heavens,
where did that come from?" Of course, a lot of it is caused by
the volcanic ash. There are many volcanoes, and you see bright
green mountains. That is from the volcanic ash that is laid all
over the ground. That is what makes for all of the big bush trees.

It is an experience, I must say, to learn what you can take,
and how you can adjust to others. I think, too, what I have
found first in my adjustment was how important food was — I
kept saying, Could I do without my own food there? How did I
know what these other foods were going to be like? I think you
really have to have an open attitude about trying, testing. The
other thing, of course, is all this asepticism with my own nursing
background. Everything has to be so clean. Well, I soon learned
that food can have some dirt and have nutritive value; this took
a while for me because I wanted to wash and I didn't have that
much water. I learned to economize, adapt.

DR. THEODORATUS: I sort of agree with that point. When I was a
child we had an old Scottish doctor who always maintained that
a little good clean dirt was good for everyone. Pull a carrot, carry
it out of the garden, simply wipe it off, and chew away on it.
Don't bother to wash it, it is good for you.

DR. LEININGER: I would also say that the way I really got close to
the people — and there are many interesting ways — was to sit

by their mu-mu's or earth ovens when they were preparing the food and eat with them there, not to isolate myself. The other thing was that as I sat out there — I was very light when I came, and, of course, they were shocked at my whiteness compared to their dark skin — they noticed the difference. But as I got browner, several times I heard them saying in their language, "Oh, you are becoming more like us." Another fascinating thing that happened was when I went to the second village. I thought I was going to be up there for a while, and I had problems with my hair — it is fine and it drops during the wet season. So I thought, why not bring one of those home permanents. I fixed my hair one night, and then I went out. There I was, very kinky and just like them. They said, "You *are* one of us!" So, there are ways of building relationships.

QUESTION: How about the language? Did you have an interpreter or did you learn the language?

ANSWER: (Dr. Leininger) The language of these people was not recorded, and this presented some problem, but before I went to New Guinea I did the summer school linguistics study and was able to record and learn the language. What I did the first two or three weeks, I really was curious about non-verbal communication, so I was in the right position to study it. I had to learn the language, and fortunately, there was one boy in the community who could speak English, and he was interested in working with me, thank goodness. That helped a lot, and it moved my progress along quite rapidly.

But I was very glad that I did study the language because there are so many things in food and even in feelings. I studied quite a bit in depth about their psychological make-up. Some things vary; for instance with anger, there are about five different varieties of anger. So it was very important that I got the different kinds of anger. I did the same with foods. To really make a good study of them, one must know the language. I never became really proficient, but I learned enough that I could do some testing and interviewing.

In the second village I could not bring my interpreter because he was a traditional enemy, and I couldn't have an enemy in the village. I was enough. I managed, and I think it really forced me to move right along. What I would do is jot down things if I wasn't certain about them, and then I would check with him later on. There were a few dialect differences because one was close to the border, but language can be a big, big barrier.

The other thing I found after I was there was a tonal language. There are not too many tonal languages in the world, except in Africa. This was another problem where I had to go back and re-work some of the material I had gotten. It had the wrong meaning by tone. So, for instance, if I dropped the tone at the ending, that meant one thing. If I raised my tone at the end of the statement, that meant almost the opposite. So it was different.

QUESTION: What, if any, benefit will ever accrue from these people being studied?

ANSWER: (Dr. Leininger) I think to begin with, there is the very basic knowledge that we are talking about — just to understand people. I think they do serve as the springboard for the introduction of change in terms of the people themselves. This was a question. As the people were revealing more intimate knowledge to me they generally asked questions about whether they would ever see what I had done. The people in both villages were just beginning to start a school, a little one-room school. What I said to them was that I hoped that someday some of this information they could get back, and I do plan to write a small booklet, particularly for the children, on their way of life. I think it could come back to them.

Another thing I think at this point is how valuable this information is to other people working with them and using the material. It is very valuable. I think another thing, also, that comes out is more in one's experience with persons from another culture. I think that there is much education, many interests that are exchanged between the two. But it is in ethnography too, that one has to watch that he doesn't start to change their attitudes right away or he will not get some good basic material that they want to reveal to him. They may be too eager to please the outsider, to say what he wants them to say rather than what they really want to say. I think probably, I certainly hope, that I can get back someday. I perhaps could be of more help to them the next time because I was truly a learner in this situation.

QUESTION: I would like to ask in relationship to that, how well do you feel information like yours that you gathered is being used by the World Health Organizations that dispense food, and people like those who give goats when they are not needed and so forth?

ANSWER: (Dr. Leininger) I really think that first of all it is my own fault. I haven't really taken the material on nutritional needs and put it together so they can use it. It begins, first of all, with me. I should really get some of this material out as fast as I can so that it would be available. The second thing, I think, is really trying to stimulate these people to use it. Sometimes they have not. It is left sitting there. Sometimes they are not even aware that people have been into their country and have this information.

This is another problem — how can we communicate to others that this is available? I hope that it will be used. I think there is a bit more sensitivity in Washington, but I will see what my other colleagues say, about beginning to use more anthropological material. I think in our educational systems much more is being done in the use of materials like this, but I think we still can have more open discussions and really work for the use of the material. Some places are not using it, I must say, only very limitedly. Dr. Lang might like to comment. He came in with me this morning from the University of Colorado, and he has done quite a bit of work in Africa. He would be a good person also to have on one of your programs in the future, as he is interested in the nutritional needs of people.

DR. LANG: I would like to address myself to the question of what good does it do for the people. I think there are really two aspects to this, one of which is, it may not do any good directly to the people, what Dr. Leininger has done in New Guinea. However, the Australians, for instance, in whose administrative area they are located, have to make decisions about what to do, where to put their efforts, and it has become very important to them to make decisions in which this kind of knowledge, what they do now, becomes very revelant. It means allocation of resources about, let us call it guided social and cultural change in which, if they do not have any knowledge or prior knowledge about the people with whom they are dealing, they must make, pretty much, stabs in the dark.

The second point is that much of this knowledge is very important; as Dr. Leininger pointed out, there are tremendous gaps in our knowledge about how people respond to food. This especially refers not only to cultural differences but also to universals in food habits. If we had known more, for instance, right after the war about lactase deficiency, we would not have sent so much powdered milk to several populations around the world, and we would have had more success that we did have. The same thing is true in India and in East Africa particularly. We know that even small population clusters respond differently to this, and we don't have enough knowledge to decide what should be done. For instance, among the people in East Africa, should we push them to become dairy farmers? Well, they can't consume milk themselves for there are no refrigeration facilities available to them. That would be very foolish, to push this aspect of the development program. It becomes very important, it seems to me, for development planning.

FOOD HABITS IN NON-INDUSTRIAL SOCIETIES

FRANK W. MOORE

Human Relations Area Files, Inc.

New Haven, Conn.

INTRODUCTION

The data presented in this paper were collected in 1962-64 during the course of a project sponsored by the Quartermaster Corps for the purpose of describing and recording the food habits and preferences of the native peoples of South and East Asia, Oceania, the Middle East, Africa, and Latin America. This paper pertains entirely to those areas, and does not deal with Europe, North or Central Asia, China, or North America (north of Mexico).

Data were collected on a total of 383 societies. No effort was made to select a sample of cultures beyond achieving a general geographic balance. Information was gathered as available. The literature on several hundred additional societies was examined but not included in the final report because of inadequacy of reporting, unreliability, or because it pertained to the period before 1930. The base line for the study was 1950, but older material (to 1930) was used in some cases. All but 35 of the societies covered were surveyed from the literature. The 35 exceptions were the result of questionnaires sent to field workers or interviews conducted by staff members of HRAF.

The research design of a project of this size was a major problem. Approximately 500,000 separate items of information (data on 38 different aspects of an average of 35 foods for each of 383 societies)

This paper is based on Vol. I, Part 1 of the *Food Habits Survey* Final Report, Project No. 7X84-06-032. New Haven, 1964.

had to be collected in a uniform format suitable for machine process-ing. To this end a series of data collection sheets was developed (Illustrations 1-3).

Obviously the specific findings of a project of this magnitude can-not be presented in this brief report. Presented below are the results of the general area surveys and a concluding section on statistical and other findings of the study over all.

The following surveys give a view of the general background and specific nature of the relationships between culture, environ-ment, and food patterns in major areas containing a number of ethnic units.

The surveys are arranged from west to east, starting with Africa:

1. Sub-Saharan Africa
2. The Middle East
3. The Indian Subcontinent
4. East Asia
5. Southeast Asia
6. Austral-Oceania
7. South and Middle America

The major area groupings have been devised on the basis of broad cultural, ethnic, geographical, and economic factors and coincide with previous cultural unit breakdowns to only a limited degree.

SUB-SAHARAN AFRICA

Indigenous peoples in this region, in general, tend to be mal-nourished. That is, in many cases the quantity of food ingested is adequate, but quality is lacking. Much of the population depends upon a single staple, which forms as much as 75 to 80 percent of the caloric intake, with the result that adequate quantities of vitamins, minerals, and other nutrients are not ingested. As a result of these deficiencies, chronic liver disease, hyper susceptibility to infectious disease, and low vitality are common and destructive facts of every-day life.

Hunting and gathering survive today as the mainstay of exis-tence only among a few remnant peoples, such as the Bushmen, the Bambuti, and the Dorobo. As a subsidiary means of subsistence,

CULTURAL BACKGROUND DATA FORM
ILLUSTRATION I (Reduced)

1. IDENTIFICATION			2. LOCATION					3. DEMOGRAPHY	
M D △ 1		1	N 3 6 E/W △ 3 7 △ △ △ △ △ 9	1 9 5 4				△ △ △ △ △ 3 2 6	△/✓
T OWC Number Sub No.	Latitude	Longitude	Min. Alt.	Max. Alt.		Year of Census	Total Population		

Names & Information Area	Nation Syria	Trends & Comment
Tell Toqaan : A small moslem Arab farming village community in the north-west plain area of Syria. Population is made up of traditional peasants and of recently sedentrized pastoralists all belonging to the Sunni sect of Islam. The settled peasants in village represent forteen different tribal affiliation. Besides this Arab population there are few foreign families i.e Circassian, Kurds and Turkish . 1:25-27	Division Range & Area Village of Tell Toqaan lies at one of lowest points of a minor inland drainage basin in NW quarter of Syria. Average alt of land is 255 m. and it lies on shallow water table (water begins to show at average level of 6-8 ft. of digging.) Land is one of most fertile in area. 1:17 2608.62 aws.	Total population of Syria in 1960 was 4,561,000 majority of whom are rural farmers. UN Demographic Book 56 families live at Tell Toqaan and total population is 326. Besides these there are few nomadic families that camp certain seasons in vicinity of village. 1:22

4. FOODS
    In Tell Toqaan as in all the Middle East, economic status determines the quality and quantity of food consumed. The wealthier having a more varied diet with regular consumption of meats and fruit. The year round staples of diet of average consumer in the village are: wheat cooked in various ways in addition to bread, onions and garlic, lentils, clarified butter, yoghurt and tea. Dates and cheese are consumed in larger amounts by people of pastoralist tradition than the real peasants. Most of the food is boiled in water yoghurt or meat, and very few are fried in olive oil or ghee. 1:127
    Meat is an infrequent item of the diet and is usually served at special occasions when entertaining or celebrating. Animals that die naturally are never used for food, since an animal has to be ritually butchered. There is a rumour that the Circassian (a foreign minority in village) eat horse meat but the Arabs do not. Brain and tongue of animal are considered delicacies and the internal organs are usually given to the children to roast and eat. 1:105-107
sugar molasses & tea - daily consumed.
    No alcoholic beverages are drunk in village; the landlords however consume arak: licorice flavored drink and beer and other imported hard liquors. 1:129 rejected meats: poate and rabbit.

5. COMBINATIONS Main dish is burghul ie cracked wheat cooked with clafified butter, onions and garlic. At times lentils are added to the dish and in poorer households maize. 1:129
    Another dish made only occasionally and considered treat is libii : After goats and sheep give birth, the female animal gives sugma rather than milk; a little of this is milked from each animal and cooked with sugar and butter into a sweet custard like dish called libii. 1:102

6. ORIENTATION
    Before eating, each member of family recites prayer of thanks. Bread is an item of food that requires special treatment and respect. If some is found on floor it is to be picked up immediatly, held to forhead and eaten. 1:132

7. HABITS A light breakfast of bread and tea is eaten on rising. Lunch is usually eaten in field between ten and twelve and consists of bread, onions and leftovers. main meal is served after sunset. Men and older sons are served first and leter women and small children. People sit around a circular mat on which the dishes and pots are placed. They eat with the aid of bread and using the right hand only. If guests are present, then they sit at table and serve with various utensils. 1:128

8. CHANGE
    Tea is recent introduction and because of its cheapness it has become very popular replacing coffee. 1:128 accepted introduction: conned beef (us park) canned milk, conned peaches, conned pears - rejected conned pineapple.

9. NUTRITION
    Population presents appearance of hardy people, once childhood is survived. There are though some noticable congenital and functional disabilities. Malaria is endemic in village, respiratory illnesses are chronic and many complaints of gastrointestinal nature. 1:23

10. ANTHROPOPHAGY	11. NARCOTICS	12. CONTAINER
Historic ☐ Pres. Ni info, ☐ Abs. Current 1:(1) ☐ Pres. ☐ Abs.	Tobacco smoking. 1:142	tinned hand-beaten copper pots and pans, imported aluminum utensils, wooden and metal spoons. Glass and chinaware. 1:129,130

however, hunting and gathering retain some importance over most of Africa. Fishing is practiced as a subsidiary economic pursuit where geographical conditions permit. In only a few societies, however, is fishing the dominant activity, and then generally only where the environment does not permit agriculture or animal husbandry as the major industry.

FOOD DATA QUESTIONNAIRE
ILLUSTRATION II (Reduced)

FS5R1   HRAF FOOD STUDY QUESTIONNAIRE

YOUR NAME _Louise E Sweet_ Culture _Tell Tognan. Syrian Muslim farming village_

Common name of source and/or Binomial _Wheat_

Native name of source _HunTa_

Common name of foodstuff ~~wheat~~ _cereal, grain, seed_ ? Native name of foodstuff ___

1. Is the foodstuff: obtainable throughout the territory of the group you are reporting on _X_ only locally obtainable___ . If generally obtainable,
is it also: abundant _X_ adequate___ scarce___ . If only locally obtainable is it at the same time: abundant___ adequate___ scarce___ .

2. Is the foodstuff: gathered, collected, or caught___ raised _X_ imported from outside the group___ .

3. Is the foodstuff: high prestige (e. g. caviar)___ low prestige (e.g. pig ears)___ variable _X_ no distinction___ . [low in the presence of rice / high ... " ... maize or barley]

4. Characterize the foodstuff (e.g. cereal, root, vegetable, milk, etc.) _ Cereal_

5. Are other uses made of the foodstuff, e.g., medicinal, ritual, stimulant, etc. _some ritual_

6. Indicate the color of the foodstuff (e.g., red, brownish, speckled grey, etc.) _light brown_

7. Is the foodstuff known to be, or thought to be toxic _No_ . If so, is it: rendered harmless by removal of the toxic agent___ counteracted by eating
in combination with some other foodstuff___ throught to be toxic only during certain periods and thus only partially avoided___ .

8. Indicate here methods of preservation or storage of foodstuff. Suggested terms: drying, smoking, salting, pickling, canning, etc.
parboiling, drying

9. Indicate the most frequent method of preparing the foodstuff for eating by writing in the numbered spaces below the successive processes in the
order in which they are undertaken. Suggested terms: boil, steam, bake, marinate, ferment, age, pound, peel, grate, mix, dry, mold. If
foodstuff is always eaten raw, indicate this on the first line. _(cracked : partially ground; very coarse)_

   1. _boiled in porridge_ 2. _ground to flour, baked_ 3. _cracked, soaked, fried_ 4. _cracked, soaked, stewed in leban_
   5.   6.   7.   8.

¬ (4 processes here with different dishes resulting. Sorry) The order is of frequency)

10. Indicate here additional or alternative methods of preparation: there is no method other than the one indicated above___ a few additional
methods___ many additional methods___ foodstuff can be eaten raw in addition to being prepared in one or more ways___ .

11. Once a foodstuff is prepared for eating it is termed a dish. Indicate below the names of the dish (e.g. pudding, stew, bread, boiled meat, etc.)
Common name of dish ①_burġl_ ②_bread_ ③ ? ④ ? Native name of dish ①_burġl_ ② _xobs_ ④ _Kibbie_ ⑤ _Kibbie_

12. Characterize, if appropriate, the reconstituted shape of the dish, e.g., loaves, balls, etc. ①_soft mass_ ②_flat round loaves_
③ _small cakes_

13. Is the dish:highly preferred _X_ _all_ preferred___ accepted readily___ disliked___ eaten only in emergency___ no preference expressed___ .

14. Is the dish consumed primarily in: urban areas _X_ rural areas _X_ upper class___ lower class _X_ special (e.g., regional) groups___
no differentiation___ .

15. Is the dish consumed by: males only___ females only___ primarily males___ primarily females___ no differentiation _X_ .

16. Is the dish consumed by: (primarily) unweaned infants _X_ children _X_ adolescents _X_ aged _X_ all but infants___ no differentiation___ .

17. Are taboos imposed on consumption of the dish? _No_ . If so, do they apply to: all of the people some of the time___ some of the people all of the
time___ some of the people some of the time___ .

18. Is the dish consumed: pretty regularly when in season___ only occasionally when in season___ pretty regularly throughout the year _X_ 1-2
only occasionally throughout the year___ on special (e.g. ritual, festivals, etc.) occasions only (specify) _X_ 3-4 (gureṭs) .

19. Indicate if possible the taste of the dish by checking one of the following: salty___ piquant___ bitter___ sour___ strong___ tasteless___
sweet-nutty _X_ other (specify)___

20. Indicate if possible the textural appearance of the dish by checking one of the following: liquid___ viscous___ soupy (lumpy)___ mashed___
gelatinous___ solid-brittle___ granular _X_ other (specify)___

21. Indicate if possible the odor of the dish by checking one of the following: spicy___ sour___ sweet _X_ foul___ mild___ odorless___
other (specify)___

22. Is the dish usually consumed: as part of a regular meal _X_ as a between meals snack___ undifferentiated___ .

23. Is the dish used as a travel food: exclusively___ occasionally _2_ never _1, 3, 4_

24. Is the dish combined with other dishes to make a more complex dish (e.g. noodles & meat to make lasagna): always___ often _2-3 4_ sometimes _1_
never___ .

Additional comments: _I've put the 4 major ways of cooking wheat here. ① Burġl and ② Bread_
are darley village fare.

FOOD DATA QUESTIONNAIRE
ILLUSTRATION III (Reduced)

Initial: A V

T	OWC	SERIAL	BINOMIAL	
	M D Δ 1 1	Δ 1 6	T R I T I C U M / A E S T I V U M	

COMMON NAME: SOURCE
W H E A T

NATIVE NAME: SOURCE
H U N T A

COMMON NAME: FOOD STUFF
S E E D * W H E A T , C R A C K E D

NATIVE NAME: FOOD STUFF
B U R G H U L

I Major Class F		II Distribution by Locality of Food Stuff		III Plentifulness (see II) of Food Stuff		IV Procurement of Food Stuff		V Prestige Value of Food Stuff	
	0	No. Info.	0	No. Info.	0	No. Info.	0	No. Info	0
Primary	1 ✕	Universally Available	1 ✕	Surplus	1	Gather	1	Very high	1
Sub-Primary	2	Generally Available	2	Abundant	2 ✕	Raise	2 ✕	High	2 ✕
Secondary	3	Locally Available	3	Adequate	3	Import	3	Medium	3
Complement	4	Not Available	4	Scarce	4	Gather-Raise	4	Low	4
Rejected	5		5	Very scarce	5	Gather-Import	5	Variable	5
Other	6		6	Non-existent	6	Raise-Import	6	No distinction	6
	7		7		7	Gather-Raise-Import	7		7
	8		8		8	Other	8		8
	9	Not Applicable	9	N.A.	9	N.A.	9	N.A.	9
VI Character of Food Stuff (A)		VII Character of Food Stuff (B)		VIII Other Uses of Food Stuff		IX Color of Food Stuff		X Number of Other Methods of Preparation of Food Stuff	
No. Info.	0	No Info.	0	No Info.	0 ✕	No Info	0 ✕	No Info.	0
Cereal	1	Fish	1	Medicinal	1	Red - Orange	1	None	1
Roots and misc. starch	2	Milk and products	2	Ritual	2	Yellow	2	Raw	2
Fruits	3	Fats, visible animal	3	Stimulant/Depressive	3	Green	3	Few	3 ✕
Sweets	4	Fats, visible vegetable	4	Medicinal-Ritual	4	Blue - Purple	4	Many	4
Legumes	5	Eggs	5	Medicinal - S/D	5	Whitish	5	Raw-few	5
Nuts	6		6	Ritual S/D	6	Brownish	6	Raw-many	6
Vegetables	7		7	All above	7	Black	7		7
Meat	8	Other	8	Other	8	Other (ot varied)	8		8
N.A.	9	N.A	9 ✕	N.A.	9	N.A.	9	N.A	9
XI Toxicity of Food Stuff		XII Main Method of Preparation A		XIII Main Method of Preparation B		XIV Main Method of Preparation C		XV Main Method of Preparation D	
No. Info.	0 ✕	No Info.	0	No Info.	0	No Info.	0	No Info.	0
Rejected	1	Cook	1	Cook	1	Cook	1	Cook Boil	1 ✕
Removed	2	Wash - Soak	2	Wash - Soak	2	Wash - Soak	2	Wash - Soak	2
Counteracted	3	Age	3	Age	3	Age	3	Age	3
Adapted to	4	Pound - Separate	4	Pound - Separate	4	Pound - Separate	4	Pound - Separate	4
Avoided periodically	5	Mix	5	Mix	5	Mix	5	Mix	5
	6	Dry	6	Dry	6	Dry	6	Dry	6
	7	Cake	7	Cake	7	Cake	7	Cake	7
	8	Other	8	Other	8	Other	8	Other	8
N.A.	9	N.A.	9 ✕	N.A.	9 ✕	N.A.	9 ✕	N.A.	9
XVI Preservation of Dish F		XVII Reconstituted Shape of Dish		XVIII Overall Acceptability of Dish		XIX Demographic Differentiation in Use of Dish		XX Sex of User of Dish	
No. Info.	0	No Info.	0	No Info.	0	No Info.	0	No Info.	0
Drying - Smoking	1	Flat	1	Highly Preferred	1	Urban primarily	1	Males only	1
Salting - Sugaring	2	Loaves	2	Preferred	2 ✕	Rural primarily	2	Females only	2
Freezing	3	Spherical	3	Accepted readily	3	Upper class primarily	3	Males primarily	3
Sealing	4	Sticks	4	Acceptable substitute	4	Lower class primarily	4	Females primarily	4
Pickling	5	Noodles	5	Disliked	5	Special groups primarily	5	No differentiation	5 ✕
Cooking	6	Varied	6	Variable	6	2 or more of above	6		6
Store only	7 ✕		7	No Preference	7	No differentiation	7 ✕		7
Other	8	Other	8	Other	8		8		8
N.A.	9	N.A.	9	N.A.	9 ✕	N.A.	9	N.A.	9
XXI Age of User of Dish		XXII Food Taboos on Dish		XXIII Seasonal and Daily Frequency of Dish		XXIV Taste of Dish		XXV Odor of Dish	
No. Info.	0	No Info.	0	No. Info.	0	No Info.	0 ✕	No Info.	0 ✕
Infants primarily	1	Absolute	1	Regularly in Season	1	Salty	1	Spicy	1
Children primarily	2	All people some time	2	Regularly no Season	2 ✕	Piquant	2	Sour	2
Adolescents primarily	3	Some people all time	3	Occasionally in Season	3	Bitter	3	Sweet	3
Adults primarily	4	Some people some time	4	Occasional no Season	4	Sour	4	Foul	4
Elderly primarily	5	None	5	Emergency only	5	Strong	5	Mild	5
All but infants	6 ✕		6	Special Occasions only	6	Tasteless	6	Odorless	6
All other combinations	7		7		7	Sweet - Nutty	7		7
No differentiation	8		8		8	Other	8	Other	8
N.A	9	N.A.	9 ✕	N.A.	9	N.A	9	N.A	9
XXVI Diurnal (in season) Dish		XXVII Texture of Dish		XXVIII Travel (Dish)		XXIX Dish used in Composite Dishes		XXX	
No. Info.	0	No Info.	0	No. Info.	0 ✕	No. Info.	0	No. Info.	0
Meal food	1 ✕	Liquid	1	Travel Only	1	Never	1		1
Snack	2	Viscous	2	Travel Also	2	Sometimes	2 ✕		2
Undifferentiated	3	Soupy (lumpy)	3 ✕		3	Seldom	3		3
	4	Mashed	4		4	Often	4		4
	5	Gelatinous	5		5	Always	5		5
	6	Solid-Brittle	6		6		6		6
	7	Granular	7		7		7		7
	8	Other	8		8		8		8
N.A	9	N.A.	9	N.A.	9	N.A.	9	N A	9

COMMON NAME: DISH
G R U E L

NATIVE NAME: DISH

Reference:
Δ Δ 1   1

Animal husbandry as a subsistence activity — not counting the raising of dometicated species which contribute but slightly to the food supply — includes pigs, goats, sheep, cattle, and camels. All of these animals were introduced to the continent from Asia by way of Egypt. The goat, the most widespread of African domestic animals, except for the dog, has in many places penetrated even the tropical forest. Sheep are not used for their wool but rather for their flesh and fat tails. The cattle represent a variety of crosses between the zebu (*Bos indicus*) and Mediterranean cattle (*Bos taurus*). While cattle are widespread, they have penetrated the tropical forest zone only to a very limited extent and are excluded from many places by the presence of the tsetse fly. Cows, goats, and camels are milked throughout the area, and over most of it butter is made — for cosmetic purposes, at least, if not for food. There are a number of purely pastoral societies in Sub-Saharan Africa, mostly in East Africa.

Agriculture is practiced everywhere in Sub-Saharan Africa except among the surviving hunters and gatherers and a few of the exclusively fishing and pastoral peoples. Africans grow approximately nine-tenths of the cultivated plant varieties known to man. The plants that have attained the status of an outstanding staple in at least several of the societies of the subcontinent are as follows, listed roughly in order of importance:

> sorghum and pearl millet; maize (tropical forest and southern) manioc (Congo, Equatorial); yams and taro (Guinea coast, southern Sudan, Cameroons, and the Congo basin; bananas (tropical forest); rice (Madagascar, coastal West Africa, from Senegal to the Ivory Coast); eleusine (East Africa); fonio (western sudan); and, legumes, sweet potatoes, and teff (occasional).

A great deal of acculturation in food habits and kinds of food produced has taken place in the past and is taking place now. Over wide regions of Africa today, plants introduced in relatively recent years from the New World, notably manioc and maize, have attained dominant roles as staple crops. At times they are so dominant that the native traditions have no mention of the crops being introduced, and the people may insist that they are indigenous. There have been great migrations of peoples over large areas in the past, with concomitant changes in environments and the kinds of foods available. Within the twentieth century, however, there has been a tremendous increase in acculturation all over the area, with an increase in nationalism and attempts by newly-formed nations to emulate the customs of the longer-established nations in the rest of the world. A great deal of detribalization and urbanization has been going on, with the result that traditional diets and food patterns are breaking down and new ones being formed all over the continent.

Sub-Saharan Africa as a whole, excluding the Moslem populations of the Sudan, has been divided into six major areas:

West Africa: This area encompasses the non-Moslem peoples between northern Senegal on the west and southern Nigeria on the east. It includes a number of environments, which can be divided basically into three: the savannas of the Sudan, the mountain forests and grasslands, and the tropical forest areas along the coast. In the first area, grains, cotton, and peanuts are common crops, and shea butter is made from the oil found in the nuts of the shea tree. This is one of the major cattle-herding areas of Africa, though horses, sheep, goats, and other domestic animals are also kept. The same may be said in general for the second zone, although some crops common to the tropical forest zone are also grown here. The Guinea coast forms the third zone. The crops and livestock here are similar to those of the Central African areas, though yams are more important than manioc, and bananas are not grown in large quantities. Hunting and gathering groups are rare, agriculture being the predominant form of productivity, together with some fishing.

West Central Africa: This is the general area of the Congo Republics and the Cameroun Republic. In the northern part, there are temperate mountain forests and savannas; the economy is mixed agricultual and pastoral, with emphasis on cereal crops. However, the remainder of the area has relatively constant high temperatures during the year, heavy rainfall, and high humidity. Some of the densest forests in Africa are found here. The region is predominantly inhabited by agricultural peoples, who live in distinct villages or settlements and who have cleared sections of the forests for their farms. Root crops—particularly manioc, yams, and taro—are commonly grown, as well as bananas, plantains, palm fruits, and other fruits. The people keep domestic goats, sheep, chickens, and ducks. Fish also can be an important addition to the diet. Cattle and other large domestic animals are not kept, because of the presence of the tsetse fly. Small bands of Pygmy hunters and gatherers are scattered throughout the area, generally living in symbiotic relationships with the agricultural peoples.

Nilotic Sudan: This is primarily a grassland area of pastoral peoples, generally cattle-keepers. Some cereals are grown, and fishing is important in some communities. Because of its isolation, it is conservative in dietary patterns, although in the past there has been a good deal of missionary activity in the area.

East Central Africa: This includes most of what was British East Africa (Kenya, Uganda, Tanganyika, Zanzibar, Zambia), as well as the former Belgian Trust Territories of Ruanda and Urundi. The northern part is mixed agricultural and pastoral, and the southern part generally agricultural. Rainfall is moderate in these areas. The temperatures are high during the day, but drop at night. There are some pockets of tropical forest, such as the Buganda area of Uganda, where plantains and other tropical forest crops are important, but much of the region is grassland, devoted to grain crops and cattle herding. Basic foods are cow's milk, prepared in several different ways, and various forms of porridge and other prepared grains. Root crops are relatively unimportant. Small domestic animals are found, and there is some fishing in the Lakes area.

In some cases, the choice of productive activity has clearly been determined by environment; while in other cases it has been made in terms of the past interests and experience of a particular group. Cattle generally have an importance in excess of their food value in terms of prestige and trade. Some small groups of hunting and gathering peoples are found. These regions have been the scene of extensive movements of peoples, particularly pastoral peoples, often with considerable warfare.

Southern Africa: This includes Angola, Malawi, Southern Rhodesia, Mozambique, Swaziland, Bechuanaland, Basutoland, and the Union of South Africa. The region can be divided into three different environmental areas. The first is a savanna which extends through the center of the area, including the Malawi, Southern Rhodesia, part of Angola, and the Union. There temperatures remain high during most of the year. Cattle herding and grain crop farming are the chief productive techniques, while small domestic animals are also kept. The second is the desert zone in the west, consisting of the Kalahari Desert and its environs. Much of this area is flat grassland, with some bush regions. The Bushmen live in the drier areas, while the cattle-herding Hottentot and Bergdama live in the grassier areas.

The third zone has a Mediterranean environment and extends from the Cape of Good Hope northeastward to the Limpopo river region. The people of the area around the Cape grow vegetables and grain crops (wheat, barley, oats), and also herd cattle and sheep. To the northeast, the area is a high plateau, with relatively flat, dry grassland and bush country, and a subtropical coastal area. Much of the region has been taken over by European farmers, and the natives generally live on restricted reserves, with their traditional cultures greatly modified.

Madagascar (including the Comoros): The island has a climate that is extremely varied, but which can be divided into three geo-graphical zones. A rugged central plateau is relatively cool, with seasonal rainfall. Wet rice, grown in terraced fields, is the staple here. In the west and south, the plateau slopes to the sea. In these lower areas the climate is hot and dry, and open plains and bush are common. Since the soil is inadequate for agriculture, cattle herding is the main occupation. To the east of the central plateau, an escarpment region, with high rainfall and heavy forests, blends into the eastern coastal zone, which is hot and humid. In these eastern sections, maize, wet and dry rice, taro, and sweet potatoes are grown. The islanders speak mainly a single Malayo-Polynesian language, Malagasy, and many characteristics of their culture indicate extensive contact with Southeast Asia. The Comoros are a mixture of Malagasy, Negro, and Arabic elements and are mainly dependent on fishing and agriculture for their subsistence.

THE MIDDLE EAST

The term Middle East, as used here, refers to the area connecting Africa, Europe, and Asia. The predominantly Moslem nations of the region extend from Turkey in the north to the limits of the

Sudan in the south, and from Afghanistan in the east to Morocco in the west. The three exceptions to this religious and political prominence of Islam are Coptic Ethiopia, primarily Christian Lebanon, and Jewish Israel. Approximately 90 percent of the population are Moslems, 4 percent are Christians (divided among several denominations), less than 2 percent are Jewish, and another 2 percent in southern Sudan belong to African tribal cults. The rest belong to semi-Moslem sects (e.g. the Druze).

Over much of this area, the year is divided into a hot rainless period and a rainy one in which precipitation may or may not be fully adequate for raising crops. This weather has led to a system of agriculture in which "mixed" farming (the combination of cultivation and animal husbandry) has had little or no place. Farming is generally of the peasant subsistence type. Geographically, the area is characterized by a basic dichotomy between desert and arable lands. Over 90 percent of the area is desert, or at best grazing steppe, with great extremes of temperature, almost no rain, and a very scanty vegetation of low grass and drought-resistant bushes. The agricultural areas are, generally speaking, Mediterranean in character, with long, hot, rainless summers, rainy, temperate winters, and a native vegetation ranging from grass to open deciduous forests. The transition from desert to arable land is gradual, with the notable exceptions of the two zones of the Nile and the Tigris-Euphrates valleys.

The peoples of the Middle East, in their adaptations to their physical environment, largely conform to this basic dichotomy of desert and cultivated land. The deserts are the home of nomadic, animal breeding tribues. The arable land, with its very different physical conditions, is the abode of the settled village farmers. The remaining population lives in towns, which generally serve as trade centers for the surrounding areas. About 20 percent of the region as a whole is composed of urban population, about 65 percent are settled farmers, and about 15 percent are nomadic or seminomadic peoples.

The nomadic and seminomadic peoples range from none at all in Lebanon to 33 percent in Afghanistan, Jordan, and the Arabian peninsula. This economic pattern of trade, agriculture, and nomad.c pastoralism in close connection is found all over the region. Complementing this is the cultural influence of Islam. Although non-Moslem minorities exist, and Islam itself has its own schisms, the influence of a single religious system has led to a culture transcending ethnic and linguistic differences.

Living conditions vary somewhat from one tribe to another and from one settled community to the next, yet these differences seem superficial when juxtaposed with the profound differences which separate the total living conditions of each type of community from those of the others. The nomads can be divided into three major type. The first, the camel nomads, depend on the camel as their main source of livelihood, and its milk is a staple food for long periods. The second type are the seminomads, also known as cattle and/or sheep and goat herders, who occupy smaller territories and who stay nearer the villages.

The third kind of nomadism, called "transhumance" is practiced over mountain areas, most typically in the Iranian plateau. Here the tribe spends the summer in the mountains and winters in the lower levels of the plateau or in the valleys. The introduction of mechanized and organized transportation in the deserts has caused a decline in the value of camels, and political boundaries have limited the range of migrations. As a result of these changes, many camel nomads are changing to cattle and smaller livestock.

The most typical way of life in the region is that of the agricultural village. With few exceptions (for example, fishing villages in Bahrain, Hadramaut, and the Marsh Arabs), the settled villagers are subsistence farmers, with a very low standard of living. Arable land in the region is restricted, and apart from petroleum, the natural resources are few. Generally speaking, the nomads live mainly on cereals, dates, milk, and milk products. The settled farmers, for the most part, consume cereals, pulses, some fruit and vegetables, and to a lesser degree milk and milk products; meat is scarce in the diet of both groups.

Because of the lack of information based on systematic nutritional surveys, little can be said about food consumption in the region except that in wide areas there appears to be a deficiency in caloric intake. In a few others (e.g. Turkey) adequate calories are available, but nutritional imbalance is widespread and serious, with a lack of "protective foods" rich in essential vitamins and minerals. Deficiency diseases such as rickets and pellagra are widely reported. Some groups are worse off now than in the past, due to increasing pressures on the land (in Egypt especially) and the rising cost of living.

For survey purposes, the region has been divided into three major areas:

The Middle East: This refers to the non-Arabic-speaking north-eastern part, including Turkey, the Zagros range, Iran, and Afghanistan, where bread, milk products, and tea are vital parts of the diet. The more prosperous people consume more rice, meat, and vegetables. Clarified butter is the preferred fat. Mulberry, acorn, and walnut flour is used in times of shortage. Taboos are Islamic and include, blood, alcoholic beverages, and the flesh of pigs, asses, horses, and carrion eaters.

The Arab Middle East: Ranging from the true camel nomads (Rwala) to the Marsh Dwellers of southern Iraq. Broadly speaking, the basic diet is very similar to that of the group above. Bread is the staff of life and is preferred when made from wheat flour, although most people have to use the cheaper barley, sorghum, or maize flour. Rice is an important food item in Iraq and on the eastern coast of Arabia, while legumes loom large in the diet of the fellahin. Christians of Lebanon may also eat raw meat and drink arak, a distilled grape vine. The Rwala are unique in that they seem to ignore the Islamic taboos, and they are reported to eat wild pig, blood of animal, and hyenas.

North Africa, the Ethiopian Plateau, and the Sudan: The coastal strip of North Africa is inhabited mainly by Berbers (or Berber-Arab mixtures), whose economy ranges from sedentary agriculture to transhumance nomadism. In general, the diet is based on cereals, supplemented by milk, vegetables, and some meat. Olive oil is the principal fat used in cooking. Fruits (especially grapes and figs) are available in season. Cereals are eaten either in the form of bread or made into the Berber national dish, couscous.

To the southeast of this area is the Ethiopian plateau and adjacent Somaliland, inhabited by ethnically different people. The ma-

jority are farmers, although many practice secondary animal husbandry. Basic food crops are cereals (including eleusine and teff),
ensete, pulses, and oil seeds. Meat and vegetables are highly seasoned
and eaten in stew form as a side dish with bread or porridge. Only
the Amhara eat raw meat. The Cushitic-speaking Galla, Kafficho,
and Somalis reject raw meat, hippopotamus, all fish, chicken, eggs,
and both horse and donkey meat. Pork is universally taboo. Despite
the Moslem injunction against alcoholic beverages, all groups indulge
in mead and beer drinking.

The Sudan corresponds roughly to that portion of Africa north
of the Equator which is under Mohammedan influence. The Sudan
is a transitional zone between the arid grasslands and deserts in the
north and the humid savannas and forests to the south and southeast. The northern part is generally good cattle country, and groups
such as the Bororo and the Adamawa Fulani specialize in cattle
breeding. The majority of the tribes are engaged in hoe agriculture
(with secondary animal hubandry). Sorghum, millet, and maize are
the staple crop. Fishing, gathering, and some hunting supplement
the food supply.

The diet of the majority of the groups in the Sudanic zone is
fairly uniform: strachy foods are eaten in the form of paste or
porridge, with a soup or sauce containing green leaves, onions, and
salt, all highly seasoned with red pepper. In the south, red palm oil
is added; in the north, peanut oil when available. Meat is eaten
occasionally and is usually added to this basic sauce. The use of
tea, tobacco, hemp, and kola nut is widespread in the region.

THE INDIAN SUBCONTINENT

The Indian peninsula (including Pakistan and Ceylon) is clearly
marked off from the rest of Asia by a broad line of high mountains.
The only open area is in the northwestern mill region. This relative
geographical isolation had led to the development of a most complex diversified culture, held together by a loose and vague Hinduism.
In the north, Islam claims a large number of adherents. Apart from
the two great religions of Hinduism and Islam, there are numerous
enclaves of primitive tribal religions and "fossils" of ancient faiths,
such as the Jains, Parsees, Jews of Cochin, etc. This cultural and
ethnic heterogeneity is explained in part by the geographical diversity

of the subcontinent. The area can be divided into three macroregions: The Extra-Peninsular mountain wall in the far north, the Indo-Gangetic plains, and the Old Peninsula Block in the south. Ceylon, separated from India by a strait only 20 miles wide, has a marked individuality and will be treated separately.

The people of India and Pakistan are predominantly agrarian, and it is estimated that around two thirds of the population (1951: 438,000,000) live directly from the soil. Agriculture outside the Himalayan region is nearly everywhere governed by the rhythm of the monsoonal year, so that water control and distribution form one of the crucial problems of India. Despite the baffling cultural diversity of India, there is an underlying unity, since the structure of the society bears the strong impress of Hinduism, especially its famous caste system. Even groups who are outside Hinduism are influenced by caste attitudes: Indian Christians, Sikhs, some Tibetan peoples, and even Moslems retain aspects of caste.

Probably the best approach to generalizing on diet in the Indian subcontinent is by using the "community" as a unit. A "community" refers primarily to a religious division, although race, language, caste, geographical localization, and broad cultural distinctions shape them apart. The largest community is that of the Hindus: in 1941 they numbered 251 million, or 66 percent of the total population. Except for Pakistan, Kasmir, and the northeastern border areas, they are spread all over the Indian peninsula. The Hindus belong to some 3,000 castes and subcastes, and traditionally each caste prepares its own foods and eats separately. The highest caste, the Brahmans, are strict vegetarians and abstain from all alcoholic drinks. The rest abstain in general from beef (the cow being held sacred), although some very poor and low castes may eat beef occasionally. The Balahis, a low weaver caste from the Nimar District, are considered untouchable by others, since they eat beef and carrion. In general, the lower one goes down the caste ladder, the greater the likelihood that the people will consume meat. The various castes all have their own dietary taboos.

The Hindu diet is generally based on cereals (rice, wheat, millet, and barley) supplemented by legumes and a large variety of vegetables, chiefly of the pumpkin and tuber varieties. Milk and milk products are generally desired, but form luxuries for the majority. Clarified butter, vegetable oils (seeds mainly), and coconut oil are the fats used in cooking. Almost all dishes cooked by Hindus are very spicy and pungent. Rice is the staple par excellence in India, except in regions in the north, where the land and climate are unsuitable for its cultivation and where wheat, barley, taro, and white potatoes take over. Apparently white potatoes were introduced by colonial administrators and missionaries and have since become important in many parts of northern India and western Tibet.

Most Hindu communities indulge in smoking tobacco and hemp, chewing betel nut, drinking liquor, and even using opium where available. Christianity, which has found most of its converts among low Hindu castes and semi-Hinduized tribes, has banned the use of liquor and narcotics and has forbidden animal sacrifices. The latter prohibition has resulted in lower meat consumption by the villagers, since formerly animals were sacrificed regularly and eaten communally. Aside from his use of European tobacco and liquor, the Hindu is rather conservative in diet and reluctant to try new foods, especially because of the various taboos.

The second community in the Indian subcontinent comprises the Tibetan-speaking tribes, including the western Tibet border people, the Sherpas of Nepal, and the Lepcha of Sikkim. The first two groups have a common diet based on wheat and barley and largely supplemented by potatoes. Being Buddhists, they are nominally vegetarians, but most groups are not averse to eating meat of animals that die by accident or are slaughtered by others. Milk curds and butter are important in the diet, as is buttered tea. Beer and rice liquor are drunk. The Lepcha diet is more "Indian," based on rice and side dishes of vegetables, which are often spiced. They also raise domestic animals for food and eat any wild animal they can lay hands on. Beverages include tea and millet beer, and a bootleg liquor made from tree ferns.

The third community on the subcontinent are the Moslems. The majority live in Pakistan, with the rest mainly in the contested state of Kashmir. Islam made most of its converts from the lowest Hindu castes. In general, the diet is based on cereals: wheat and barley, supplemented by millet and rice. Bread, some meat stew, and a vegetable dish make up the common menu. Animals have to be slaughtered in ritual fashion to be rendered acceptable to a Moslem; the pig and its flesh are taboo, and a general fast during the month of Ramadan is observed. In general, Islam prohibits the use of alcoholic beverages.

The next group is the third largest community in India and is comprehensively labeled "tribes." This, however, is a very heterogeneous and very scattered grouping, with two major zones of concentration: the Assam-Burma Hills and the jungles of central India. The tribes are in general pagan shifting cultivators, and lately are being included in the lowest strata of Hindu society, which usually means that they have to renounce beef eating and shift to a vegetarian diet. The majority still rely on limited hunting for meat and on collecting wild roots, leaves, and fruits. Staples are again cereals, usually pounded and boiled into porridges and eaten with various curries and chutneys. Since most of the aboriginal tribes have been pushed back into more inhospitable area (the hills or jungles or both), the majority have to grow millet, Job's-tears, or tubers rather than their preferred rice. All tribes legally distill liquor, smoke extensively — both tobacco and hemp — chew betel nut, and occasionally take opium.

To sum up: The food and eating habits of the Indian subcontinent strongly reflect Hindu influences. The diet is inclined to be conservative, and, despite the fact that it is rather similar in its basic elements, it differs in the number and kinds of taboos that apply to the component castes and groups. These differences reflect the stratified social structure and serve to reinforce it.

Ceylon: The Island of Ceylon is essentially a detached portion of southern India, which it resembles in land form, climatic regions, natural vegetation, and soils. The dominant ethnic groups, the Sinhalese, have retained their Buddhism and have had considerable influence on Buddhists in other lands. There also exists on the island a small minority of aboriginal Australoid people, the Veddas, confined to east-central Ceylon. The island has a dual economy and plural society; the indigenous economy is centered on the cultivation of rice on irrigated land. Rice is the basic foodstuff, but is supplemented by various fruits and vegetables grown on "high" land and by grain grown by shifting cultivation. Fishing is also important. Fish, meats, and vegetables are most often served as curries with boiled rice.

Hinduism has left its mark on the theoretically casteless Buddhist soicety of the Sinhalese. Fishing is conidered a low-class occupation, labor tends to be immobile, and there are many food restrictions. Even the aboriginal Vedda have taboos that can be explained as transfers from Hinduism, such as their rejection of beef, water-buffalo, eagle, and leopard.

EAST ASIA

East Asia, separated from the Indian subcontinent on the south and west by the vast Tibetan complex of mountains and plateaus, from Southeast Asia by the mountainous border region, and from Siberia on the north by the Gobi desert, is the home of almost a third of mankind. The most densely populated areas are the fertile lowland plains of the great rivers and the coastal and mountain low-lands of South China, Korea, and Japan.

Climatically, East Asia can be characterized as having seasonal shifts in winds and precipitation. The great latitudinal spread, orographic factors, and maritime influences (especially in Japan and in island areas) determine the varied climate. The main area has a characteristic temperate zone climate, with cold winters and hot summers. The areas near the Pacific Ocean receive the bulk of their rainfall in the cooler months. The northwest is generally cold and dry, while the south coast is humid and subtropical.

The distinctive climate, together with the isolation resulting from the great mountain and desert barriers, has given East Asia an agricultural pattern that is quite different from that of the rest of Asia. Since rice grows best in flooded fields and is well adapted to the hot wet summers of this area, the yield per acre of rice is much larger than that of wheat. Thus, rice and other cereals produced from the 20 percent of East Asia's land that is arable support a heavier population than in most of Europe or West Asia.

The areas included in this study fall into the following four major groups: 1) Northeast Asia, Korea Cheju, rural Japan, and the Ryukyu Islands, 2) the Non-Han people of South China and of

3) the North and West Periphery (the Tibetans and Ainu), and 4) the Formosan aborigines. As previously mentioned, China is not included in this study.

Despite the mountainous topography, there is intensive rice farming in Northeast Asia, due to an abundant water supply and a climate that is extremely favorable for agriculture However, shortage of rice is common, and the problem is most acute in islands like Cheju and the Ryukyus. The common statement that rice is *the* staple in the East Asian diet needs re-evaluation and qualification. In most regions and among the bulk of the population, the preferred staple, steamed polished rice, is often (if not always) "stretched" by being mixed with other cereals, such as barley or millet, or with legumes or potatoes. In some areas, such as Cheju and the Ryukyus, rice is eaten only on special occasions by the vast majority of the population. Only during a few months following the harvest can the people afford rice as a significant proportion of their cereal diet, which represents almost 80 percent of their total caloric intake. Thus, cereals are the staple foods, not rice alone as is commonly assumed.

Next to ceeral foods, vegetables provide the bulk of the diet. A wide variety of both cultivated and wild vegetables are eaten throughout the year. Vegetable pickles, necessary go-along-with dishes in both Japan and Korea (but not in the Ryukyus), provide vitamins during the winter months. The popular use of noodles and soybean products, the limited use of meat, poultry, eggs, fish, and seaweed, and the lack of dairy products in the diet seem to be common characteristics of all Northeast Asian peoples. While the Japanese emphasize raw and colorful dishes and do only a minimum of cooking, Koreans use more spices and have developed more elaborate cooking methods. Tea drinking is part of Japanese diet as well as a ritual, but Koreans use little tea.

The culturally diverse people settled in the highlands of the southwestern provinces of China, and in the northern regions of Southeast Asia, live in relative isolation and have developed numerous cultural variations in the course of their adaption to the local altitude, climate, and to the neighboring dominant cultural groups. They share a common hostility toward the dominant Han or Thai. They may be classified under at least three subheadings: the Miao, the Yao, a third group made up of the Lolo, Lisu, and Monguor.

The Miao, further subdivided into the Red, Black, Blue, White, Flowery, and other groups, were estimated at about 2,700,000 people in 1953. They are found in Kweichow and its neighboring provinces and in North Vietnam, Laos, and northern Thailand. Some groups eat maize porridge, while others have glutinous rice as their major staple. However, both maize and glutinous rice seem to be used by all groups either as a primary or as a subprimary foodstuff. Sour dishes and pickled vegetables are common, and red pepper is the most important condiment. The use of animal blood for food, the scarcity of meat, and the popularity of betel nut chewing seem to be common denominators.

The Yao, less numerous than the Miao, are estimated at about 800,000, of which 660,000 live in mainland China. They are dispersed throughout Hunan province, Hainan, Indochina, and northern Thailand. Some cultivate irrigated rice, while others engage in slash-and-burn techniques of shifting cultivation suitable to their environment. Nonglutinous rice is the major staple, supplemented by maize and tubers. Unlike some Miao groups, neither maize nor tubers are primaries, but are eaten only as supplementary foods. Hot peppers and sour foods are also popular among the Yao. Meat is eaten only on special occasions. Widespread consumption of rice wine and some use of opium are recorded, but there is no account of betel chewing. The so-called "Hainen Miao" are considered by some authorities to be Yao from a linguistic point of view, and their food habits support this hypothesis. The Miao of Hainan, unlike other Miao people, eat rice gruel and do not like maize.

The third subgroup in terms of their food patterns are the Lolo and Lisu, together with the Lahu and Akha of the Tibeto-Burman linguistic group. The Monguor diet also seems to fall into this pattern. This subgroup is found throughout the mountainous areas of Yunan, extending north into southwestern Szechwan, east into western Kweichow, and south into northern Indochina. The Lisu claim their original homeland to be the north, in the direction of Tibet, and their food patterns reflect some Tibetan influence.

The diet of the Lolo of China is characterized by buckwheat cakes and porridge, supplemented by vegetable soup, which may contain chicken. The Lolo of the Southeast Asia mainland eat rice and a kind of curry with vegetables. Meat is rare and eaten only on special occasions. The Lisu diet seems to be similar to that of Lolo.

The Monguor, known as Tujen or aborigines to the Chinese, comprise another non-Han group of people who share similar food habits with the Lolo. They live on the border of Kansu and Ching-hai provinces in the westernmost part of China. Like Tibetans, they prefer tea and barley (rather than buckwheat) porridge as staples, supplemented by some vegetables. Meat, together with milk products, was once the staple food, but has now become a luxury.

Among the predominantly cereal-eating people of East Asia, the Tibetans and Ainu are the only people who consume a considerable quantity of meat (or fish), milk, and milk products, with little or no vegetables. Although geographically separated — Tibet in the northwesternmost part of East Asia and the Ainu in the north of Japan, in the eastern corner of this area — the two peoples have a common ecological situation, including extreme cold. Despite the Tibetans' religious prohibition against eating meat and in spite of the Japanese effort to assimilate the Ainu to cereal culture, a high proportion of protein intake in the form of meat and dairy products can still be seen in both areas. Hot liquids, in the form of tea or soup, which accompany the cereal porridge (for the Tibetans barley, and for the Ainu, millet) are also characteristic. When available, wild plants are preferred to cultivated vegetables as food.

The mountain tribes of Formosa, closely allied to Indonesians in ethnic type, language, and culture, dwell in three different habi-tats — temperate, subtemperate, and subtropical zones — with vary-ing temperatures due to latitude and altitude. They subsist on Italian millet, rice, sweet potatoes, and taro, supplemented by meat and fish. The tribes who dwell in the temperate or subtemperate zone depend primarily on cereals and secondarily on tuber or root crops; whereas the reverse is true among those in the subtropical or tropical zone. Millet gruel or millet and other cereals mixed is their staple dish.

Pigs are found among all tribes, and chickens and domestic fowl are lacking only among the Yami of Botel Tobago Island. The Yami are linguistically and culturally more akin to the Batanese of the northern-most Philippine Island than to the rest of the Formosan aborigines. Unlike the rest of this group, the Yami do not smoke or drink, and they domesticate wild fowls. Salt is very scarce among all the Formosan aborigines.

To sum up, the diet of East Asia in general is high-carbohydrate, moderate-protein, and low-fat diet. The use of rice in combination with other cereals, plus a fair amount of legumes and vegetables, a limited amount of meat, poultry, fish, and eggs, the limited use of vegetable oils for cooking, and a lack of dairy products, seem to characterize the East Asian diet. Unlike India or the Middle East, there are few food taboos or class or caste differences in relation to food consumption. Geographic, economic, and seasonal factors seem to be the major variables of the East Asian food pattern.

Although many new foods, such as soft drinks, sweets, coffee, canned milk, etc., have been introduced to East Asia, especially during and since World War II, the basic diet seems to be un-affected. Unlike Western societies, dessert is not a part of the regular meal, though the drinking of cereal wine and the smoking of tobacco seem to be enjoyed by most of the people in East Asia, especially men and older people.

SOUTHEAST ASIA

Southeast Asia is here defined to include Upper Burma on the west, most of the former French Indo-China, and Malaya.

Historically, Southeast Asia has been a zone of convergence for Indian and Chinese cultures and a bridge between the European West and East Asia. The pressure of long-continuing Chinese expansion has caused the migration of many East Asians southward and brought about an enormous variety of ethnic, linguistic, and religious differences. Climatically, Southeast Asia can be characterized by its wet summers and dry winters. High temperatures (which vary little throughout the year), and abundant rainfall (which varies radically from season to season and from place to place) make most of Southeast Asia, except for some highland regions, a year-round growing area.

About 60 percent of the land is still in forest and woodland in an area running north-south across the continental countries to the Malay Peninsula, but there are also some agricultural regions:

the Irrawaddy central dry zone and delta, the lower Chao Phya basin, the Cambodian flats and Cochin-China delta of Tonkin, and the lower courses of innumerable lesser streams.

The people of Southeast Asia range from migrant food gatherers and hunters in the jungles to subsistence farmers in the plains. About three-fourths of the total working population is engaged in agriculture, fishing, or in elementary forest exploitation. Only 8.5 percent of the total area is under cultivation. About 60 percent of the cultivated area is devoted to rice, with 12 percent in maize and 4.3 percent in root crops, such as manioc, sweet potatoes, and yams.

Generalizations about food habits can be made in the following different patterns, corresponding roughly to the three levels of agricultural development: 1) hunting and gathering people of the Andaman Islands and the aborigines of Malaya, 2) indigenous mountain people who are engaged in shifting agriculture, and 3) sedentary rice cultivators. The last group may be again subdivided according to their staple food into a) glutinous-rice eaters and b) nonglutinous-rice eaters. Among the nonglutinous-rice eaters there seem to be two patterns of diet, one based on those who received Indian influence and consume curry dishes in quantity, and the other based on those in the southeastern corner of the continent, where curry is rare as a condiment.

Among people in Southeast Asia who obtain most of their food by collecting edible wild plants, and by hunting and fishing, are the Negrito Semang of the Malay Peninsula and the Onge and Andamans of the Andaman Islands. While the Andamans and Onge utilize meat and fish, the Semang are gatherers of wild plants and are largely vegetarians. The Andamans and Onge eat wild pigs and marine turtles as their staple foods. Insects, some wild yams, and some wild roots supplement their diets. Salt is very scarce and is considered undesirable. The Semang and Semai of Malay are gatherers who subsist primarily on wild plants, especially roots and tubers. The Semang have intimate knowledge of edible plants and have developed elaborate techniques of food preservation and of processing poisonous substances for food.

On the higher slopes and ridges away from the damp valleys and in the relatively isolated communities along the borders of India,

Pakistan, and Burma, as well as in other mountainous areas of Southeast Asia, shifting cultivation provides upland rice, millet, and Job's tears. Hunting and gathering supplements these agricultural products. In these areas, where soils are poor and the rate of soil erosion high, cereals are the major staples, supplemented by yams. The amount of rice consumed in these regions seems to be negligible in terms of the total food intake. Meat of both wild and domesticated animals is highly valued, but is scarce and consumed only during feasts and on special occasions. Curry varies in importance from group to group. The use of insects, sago palms, and wild root crops is noteworthy. Bananas and coffee are also cultivated and are used either as food or cash crops.

By far the most important grain for both shifting and sedentary cultivators in Southeast Asia is rice. A remarkably large number of district varieties of cultivated rice may be found, but the two major classes are upland or dry rice and lowland or wet rice. The cultivation of wet rice requires a more sophisticated technique and much more water than dry rice. Glutinous rice and nonglutinous varieties also require different conditions of growth. Thus the staple cereal of the people on the Southeast Asian mainland seems to be either one or the other rice, but seldom both.

In summary, the people of Southeast Asia depend primarily on rice, fish, and curry. The proportion of wild roots, tubers, animals, and insects in their total food intake seems to be greater than in Northeast Asia, although the degree to which collecting, hunting, and fishing contributes to the food supply varies with the seasons and among different people.

Cattle do not fit well into the ecology of Southeast Asia nor into the religious tradition of the people. Buddhists and Hindus do not eat beef, Moslems will not eat pork, and the native believers in animism have similar inhibitions about their totemic animals. Buffalo and small oxen, which serve primarily as draft animals, seem to be the only source of domesticated meat supply.

Fish, which supplies calcium, iodine, and salt as well as animal protein, has always been an important item, second only to rice. The emphasis on fresh water fishing rather than on deep sea fishing and the utilization of fish paste and fish sauce are unique features of this region.

Their use of chilies and sesame seeds as condiments is similar to the Chinese and other Northeast Asian people, but the use of curry is an Indian influence. The popularity of noodles among almost all the people in Southeast and Northeast Asia may be attributed to Chinese influence, and potatoes are regularly used in their curries. Corn is used more and more frequently, both as a vegetable and as a snack. Rice consumption per capita increased during the past century but the opposite trend has been evident during the present century.

AUSTRAL-OCEANIA

In terms of distances, Austral-Oceania is an extremely large area with, however, a relatively small land mass. In addition to the continent of Australia, there are thousands of islands, ranging in size from New Guinea and Borneo, among the largest in the world, down to bits of palm-covered coral, only a few acres in extent. There are three kinds of Pacific (or tropical) islands: the volcanic peak or range, surrounded by a coral reef; the coral mass, which has been thrown up to a height of a few hundred feet and is surrounded by a coral reef; and the atoll, which is simply a low coral reef, circular in shape, enclosing a lagoon instead of a land mass, and with a series of palm-covered islets.

The native ecologies are based generally, with the exception of Australia, on cultivation, but no grain crops are indigenous to the Pacific. The natives have relied mainly on root vegetables such as taro and yams, and on sago, breadfruit, bananas, and, particularly in the eastern Pacific, on the coconut. In recent years, there has been a definite trend away from taro, the traditional root crop — and to a lesser extent from yams — toward manioc and sweet potatoes. A reason for this trend is that there are more calories gained per acre from manioc and sweet potatoes. Furthermore, manioc in particular needs no storage, since it can be left in the ground until needed. This trend is found all over the area, but it is particularly noticeable in Polynesia

In French Polynesia, there is in most areas an almost total rejection of the traditional economy. Commercial fishing, plantation agriculture, and the production of copra has taken over. Most of the food (between 80 and 90 percent) is imported. Gardens are totally neglected, especially when copra prices are high. Fishing is an important activity on the smaller islands and in the coastal regions of the larger ones, where fish are frequently exchanged with inland peoples for vegetable produce.

For this study, the Pacific has been divided into five major areas: Indo-Pacific, Australia, Melanesia, Micronesia and Polynesia.

Indo-Pacific: This area might be further divided into two major subareas: Indonesia and the Philippines. In physical features and in vegetation, the Indo-Pacific area is imilar to the other Pacific areas, but its cultures are very closely allied to Asia. For many centuries the area has been affected by religious, political, and economic influences from India and China and from various European nations (Spanish, Dutch, American, and Portuguese). The cultures range from those of nomadic hunters and gatherers (particularly in Borneo) to highly developed native states ruled by rajahs and sultans. Most of these groups are agricultural, with rice the common crop, although maize, manioc, sweet potatoes, and fish are also highly important.

The Indonesian subarea consists mainly of the Republic of Indonesia, along with the portions of Malayia located on the island of Borneo. It does not include West Irian (western New Guinea). This is the area generally known as the East Indies, that group of islands from the Sulu Sea southward terminating at the eastern end of Weber's Line, west of New Guinea. This region is one of similar but widely dispersed ethnic groups.

The great majority are Malayans in physical type, with some occasional Negrito populations. Some 80 to 90 percent of the peoples are Moslems, which accounts for the absence of pork in the area. There are a large number of Christians, some Hindus, and a number of pagan tribes. The main crops are dry and wet rice, maize, manioc, soy bean, peanuts, and sweet potatoes. Fishing is important, since fish is the favorite protein food of the inhabitants. Fish are also raised in ponds.

The Philippine subarea consists of the Republic of the Philippines (population estimated at around 21,000,000). There are more than 7,000 islands in the area, but most of the land area of 115,600 square miles is concentrated in a few large islands, mainly Luzon and

Mindanao. There is a far greater range of environments in this area than in Indonesia, since the area generally runs from north to south, rather than from east to west, as in Indonesia. There is, therefore, a difference in seasons, rainfall patterns, and temperatures.

Though the vast majority are from closely related cultures, there is a diversity of race and cultures in the islands. There are some Negroid and Veddoid remnant populations, but most of the rest are Malayan in background. In terms of religion, there are three main groupings: pagans in the interior of the larger islands, Christians in the northern islands, and Moslems in the southern islands. Therefore, there is a variety of concomitant dietary patterns. For social reasons, agriculture aiming at both food and trade has become more commercialized in the Philippines than elsewhere, and maximum return, rather than sustained return, has been the farming objective. Double cropping is common.

The staple food of the whole area has generally been understood to be rice, but in the central Philippines, maize has taken its place, and root crops are perhaps more significant in caloric terms. Rice is still the preferred food in most places. Yams, sweet potatoes, and manioc are vital to the local diet and are very widely grown. Large quantities of legumes and savory or peppery vegetables are cultivated. Most of the population is vegetarian by obligation rather than by religious conviction. The chief source of animal protein is fish from inshore fishing, which is consumed exclusively in the local trade. In some areas, the collecting of wild foods is important. Animal husbandry is negligible, except for draft animals, such as zebu and carabao.

Australia: The Australian environment is so stringent that, aboriginally, probably only about 300,000 people lived in this huge area. The eastern and southeastern coasts are temperate and well drained, and the same is true for a small area on the southwestern coast. Melville and Bathurst Islands and parts of the northern coastline have a subtropical and tropical environment, but most of the rest of the continent is unproductive bushland or desert.

The Autralian aborigines constitute a separate racial stock. They were exclusively hunting and food-gathering people and were absolutely dependent on what nature produced without any assistance on their part. This still holds true for a large part of the interior, although in other areas contact with white Australians has changed the situation.

There are now about 50,000 full-blooded aborigines and about 30,000 mixed-bloods left in Australia, in addition to those who have been sumberged in the white population.

Melanesia: This area includes New Guinea and the arc of islands to the northeast of Australia extending southward as far as New Caledonia and eastward to Fiji. The Fiji Islands are transitional between Melanesia and Polynesia. The native population is about 1,700,000. Melanesia is the major home of the Oceanic Negroids, and it presents a wide variety of cultures. Widely varying percentages of racial components and isolated environments have resulted in great racial and cultural complexity, with "pygmy" peoples living in the interior of the island of New Guinea and tall-statured peoples scattered around the area as a whole.

The people are mainly sedentary agriculturalists, their principal cultivated plants being taro, yams, bananas, breadfruits, and coconuts, all Asiatic in origin. Rice is now imported and eaten by islanders with great relish. Pig raising is generally a major occupation, and fowl and dogs are also raised.

There is in most places in Melanesia a distinction between "beach" natives and "bush" natives: the former usually have wider contacts, more advanced technologies, richer diets, and consequently better physiques than the latter. Melanesia in general is one of the great disease areas of the world, with the following taking a great toll in lives and health: malaria, respiratory diseases, dysentery, framboesia, yaws, tropical ulcer, hookworm, filariasis, and beriberi. During and following World War II, there was a tremendous amount of contact with Western culture and a consequent acculturation to many new patterns, particularly in western Melanesia.

Micronesia: The hundreds of islands of Micronesia are scattered over an ocean area larger than the United States, but they contain altogether only 1,260 square miles of land area. Aboriginally, they may have contained a population of over 200,000, but in 1938 the population estimate was only 103,000. At that time the population was expanding again from a low reached around 1900. Furthest north are the Mariana Islands, the northernmost of which is near Japan. South of these islands lie the several Caroline Island archipelagoes. To the east are the atoll archipelagoes of the Marshall Islands and the Gilbert Islands.

Throughout the area most of the people earn their living by farming and fishing. The staple plant foods on the high islands are taro, breadfruit, yams, coconut, and pandanus kernels. On the infertile atolls, plant foods are scarce, and the inhabitants depend on the sea to survive.

Polynesia: The Polynesian islands are those roughly east of longitude 180° and also including New Zealand. The Hawaiian Islands to the north, though Polynesian, are not included in this survey. Easter Island is the easternmost Polynesian island. There are western Polynesian outliers in the area generally regarded as Melanesia, notably Tikopia and Ontong Java. In spite of widespread similarities in race and language, a considerable variety of cultures are found in Polynesia, some of which are correlated with environmental differences.

Nearly all the Polynesians were farmers and fishermen, although in recent years in some areas, particularly French Polynesia, the traditional economy has been rejected. For many years, taro, yams, bananas, and coconuts were the principal crops, but recently taro and yams have been supplanted in many islands by manioc and sweet potatoes, as has been noted above. Pigs, dogs, and fowl are kept wherever there is enough food for them, and these animals are used to supplement the vegetable diet. Fishing is a regular vocation, as well as a sport. Most fish, including shellfish of all kinds, are obtained in streams and lagoons and along the reefs, but the islanders also take their boats far offshore to capture tuna and bonito.

The area as a whole is highly acculturated since it has been in continuous contact with Western culture since the eighteenth century. There has, therefore, been a definite change in the dietary patterns away from the aboriginal, and most islands are dependent on trade for at least some of their foods.

SOUTH AND MIDDLE AMERICA

Most of the population of this area is ethnically mixed. Although essentially Amerindian, some European ancestry, generally Spanish or Portuguese is common over much of this area. As a concomitant of this racial and cultural mixture, there is also a mixture of food habits, dietary patterns, cultural conditioning, and actual foods cultivated. The basic starch-staples of native America-maize, bitter and sweet manioc, and potatoes — are still being grown and used, but in many areas, food staples from the rest of the world have been accepted as well. As an extreme, for the Toba, a primitive group in the northern Gran Chaco, the staple food is now macaroni and spaghetti, which is bought at trading posts in the neighborhood. There are, of course, places of interior Amazonia where only native staples are still in use, but such unmixed economies are very rare.

The Americas south of the Tropic of Capricorn have been divided into six major areas.

Middle America: This area includes the agricultural peoples from the north of Mexico to Panama. Maize remains the staple in the highlands of Mexico and Guatemala, along with beans and chili peppers. In the lowlands there is generally a mixed economy based on maize and manioc. The Seri of northern Mexico are an exception, being nonagricultural.

The Northern Lowlands: These South American lowlands contain a mixture of tropical forest and savanna grasslands. The native inhabitants are generally strongly influenced by the cultures of the Andean highlands and/or those of the tropical forests. The major staples are again maize and manioc, with bananas and plantains forming an important adjunct in many areas. Wild game and fish are also important in some places. The lowlands of Colombia, Venezuela, southern Panama, and the Guianas are included. Parts of interior lowland Colombia, however, are included with the Amazonian area. The Guianas are further distinguished by having a large proportion of East Indian and Negro inhabitants, who have imposed many of their own special food habits on the neighboring natives. In addition, the white inhabitants are mainly derived from northern Europe, unlike most of the rest of "Latin" America.

Andean: This region includes those peoples living along the backbone of South America, from Colombia to Chile. The area was dominated by Inca culture in pre-Spanish days, and much of the area today is dominated by Quechua (Inca)-speaking groups. The food staples are maize and Andean (i.e. white) potato. The potato is termed "Andean" here, since it comes in many other colors as well as white.

The region may be further broken down into three subregions: North Andean (which includes Colombia and northern Ecuador); Central Andean (which includes southern Ecuador, Peru, Northern Chile, and about half of Bolivia), the homeland of the Quechua and Aymara, the largest native groups in South America; and South Andean, which includes the rest of Chile and western Argentina and is the home of the Araucanians. There is a general dichotomy between the coastal, lowland dwellers and the inhabitants of the mountains. The highland dwellers generally have potatoes as their staple, supplemented by maize and lesser indigenous cereals or pseudo-cereals, such as quinoa; while the dwellers along the coastal deserts in the center and south generally depend upon maize and other temperate crops.

Southern Lowlands: This area consists of the rest of Argentina, southern Bolivia, southern Paraquay, Uruguay, and southern and eastern Brazil (i.e. the part that is drained southward and eastward toward the Atlantic Ocean, rather than toward the Amazon). This great area is characterized generally by temperate forests and grasslands, seed agriculture (maize, various small grains), and cattle-raising (among the European inhabitants). The cultures here are generally more heterogeneous than those of the rest of South America, with, aboriginally, nomadic hunters in the south (up through the Gran Chaco), and seed agriculture and hunting as the characteristic base of the society for much of the rest of the area. The northern part of the area is now characterized generally by caboclo culture, a mixture of Indian, Negro, and Portuguese culture elements and racial stocks.

Amazonian: This area generally embraces the region drained by the Amazon river and its tributaries. It consists of most of interior Brazil, northern Paraguay, eastern Bolivia, eastern Peru, eastern Ecuador, southeastern Colombia, and a small portion of southern Venezuela. The environment in the main is tropical rain forest, with areas of gallery forest and savanna. Root crops, particularly bitter and sweet manioc, yams, and sweet potatoes, form the basis of the diet, as well as many wild fruits, maize, and the products of hunting. There is considerable acculturation of the native tribes along the main rivers, but a great part of the area is relatively untouched by Western civilization. The central and lower Amazon area has been the great rubber-producing region of Brazil, and as such has had much contact with non-Indian cultures, although this has not altered the basic dietary pattern to any extent.

Caribbean: This area includes all the islands in the Caribbean Sea. This is a very mixed area both ethnically and in terms of dietary patterns. There are almost no native Amerinds left here, and the population is a mixture of Negro, Indian, and European, with some Indonesian elements in Trinidad. The dietary pattern is similar to that of the South American northern lowlands, based principally on root agriculture in a tropical forest environment. In addition, there is a great deal of acculturation, with food imports coming from North America and Europe.

CONCLUSION

The study of 383 societies makes it possible to generalize to some extent regarding man and his food habits, although statistical treatment of these data is not warranted, due to the inadequacy of worldwide balance in the sampling.

It appears that man is definitely a carnivore by instinct but has become a vegetarian by force of circumstances. While meat of one sort or another is often the subject of religious or social taboo, it is also true that meat is nearly always the central feature of social or ceremonial meals, whenever it is available. In ordinary life too, meat is included in the daily diet to the full extent of its availability. It is precisely because of meat's desirability that it is the subject of so many sumptuary laws and taboos. Whether meat is scarce because of its desirability or desirable because of its scarcity is a moot question, but generally speaking meat resources are exploited to their full economic extent, even considering such exceptions as the well-known Hindu prohibition of beef consumption.

A somewhat surprising generalization can be made about rice, the most prominent starch-staple in this study. While rice is very often the most desired starch-staple, it is, upon closer examination, not nearly as dominant in the diet as would be expected. It should be mentioned again in this connection that China is excluded from this study. In most cases, various other types of cereals (maize, millet, etc.) are used to supplement the inadequate rice supply. Root crops of various types (potatoes, manioc, taro, etc.) frequently account for a larger total portion of the yearly caloric intake than rice, even in such traditionally rice-eating regions as the Philippines.

In a sense, rice is similar to meat in being highly desired but in short supply for much of the population of these areas. Rice, while more highly regarded and desired than maize was second to maize in numbers of occurrences, both as a primary (staple) food and (111 to 187) as a secondary food resource. Among tubers and roots, manioc (bitter and sweet — 106 occurrences) is far ahead in popularity of taro (all types — 52 occurrences), sweet potatoes (51), yams (43), and white potatoes (10) (Illustrations 4-9).

In regard to condiments, the relatively low number of occurrences (less than 50 percent) of reports of salt consumption was unexpected. Possibly this correlates with failure on the part of field workers to bother reporting this rather obvious bit of information. Thus chili pepper (Capsicum) of New World origin ranks ahead of salt in popularity (171 occurrences). Sugar is a poor third (62) as a condiment, though in general sweet foods and drinks are highly desired and it is likely that unavailability rather than desire is the determining factor in this case.

Taboos on consumption of food resources are far more heavily weighted against used of meat (415 wild, 345 domestic) than against plants (258 wild and domestic). Many of these taboos are of short duration and apply only to very limited segments of the population, e.g. pregnant women, adolescents, etc.

Eating patterns conform very closely to economic base. When the societies in the sample were classified as to number of regular meals (0 to 4 or more), it was found that all or nearly all those societies having three or four meals were agricultural or pastoral; while hunting, fishing, or gathering societies tended very strongly to no regular meals or only one regular meal. The obvious correlation between dependable food supplies and regular meals, while

ILLUSTRATION IV

PRIMARY (STAPLE) FOODS

Listed in Order of Occurrence By Classes (All Societies)

Note: Most societies have more than one primary food resource.
Primaries listed for 5 or fewer societies not included.

Acceptability scale:

1. Highly Preferred	3. Highly Acceptable
2. Preferred	4. Acceptable

		No. of Occurrences	Acceptability Level
Cereals			
Maize		171	4
Rice (undifferentiated)	134		1
glutinous	9	161	2
nonglutinous	18		1
Millet		94	4
Sorghum		68	1
Wheat		46	1
Barley		19	3
Buckwheat		9	4
Hungry rice		5	1
Cereals, misc.		71	1
Roots and Tubers			
Manioc (undifferentiated)	38		4
bitter	36	106	4
sweet	32		4
Taro, true	41		4
giant	4	52	4
pulax	7		1
Potato, sweet		51	4
Yams		43	4
Potato, white		10	4
Aboriculture			
Bananas	49		4
Plantains	35	84	4
Coconut		43	4
Breadfruit		21	4
Dates		17	1
Sago		13	4
Pandanus		11	4
Legumes & Misc. Vegetables			
Beans		29	3
Cowpeas		5	1
Peanuts		5	1
Squash		10	4
Domestic Animals			
Cows and zebus		25	1
Fowl (ducks & chicken)		9	1
Sheep		9	1
Goats		8	1
Wild Animals			
Wild animals, misc.		19	2
Fish, misc.	94	105	1
Bonito	11		1
Elephant		5	1
Turtles		5	1

ILLUSTRATION V
SECONDARY FOOD SOURCES (ALL SOCIETIES)

Listed by rank order of occurrence with acceptability ratings.

	Occurrences	Acceptability
1. Chicken (meat and eggs)	363	2
2. Squash	222	3
3. Cow (meat and milk)	196	3
4. Maize	187	3
5. Pig, domesticated	180	2
6. Goat	166	3
7. Potato, sweet	163	3
8. Banana	160	2
9. Fish (not including specified small)	159	2
10. Beans	137	2
11. Peanut	123	3
12. Sugar cane	120	2
13. Papaya	118	3
14. Rice	111	1
15. Sheep	108	2
16. Mango	107	3
17. Onion	104	2
18. Tomato	103	3
19. Coconut	98	3
20. Taro (all types)	87	3
21. Bee (honey, primarily)	86	1
22. Manioc (unspecified)	85	3
23. Pineapple	84	3
24. Yam	80	3
25. Cucumber	71	3
26. Duck (meat primarily)	67	2
27. Eggplant	66	3
28. Potato, white	66	3
29. Watermelon	66	2
30. Coffee	58	2
31. Okra	58	3
32. Tea	58	2
33. Plantain	55	3
34. Wheat	54	2
35. Cow, Zebu, female (milk primarily)	49	3
36. Orange	49	3
37. Deer	48	3
38. Cowpea	46	3
39. Palm, oil	46	2
40. Turtle (meat and eggs)	46	3
41. Cabbage	45	3
42. Baobab	44	1
43. Palm	44	3
44. Cow, Zebu (meat and milk)	43	3
45. Pea	43	3
46. Dog	42	3
47. Guava	42	3
48. Rat	42	2
49. Breadfruit	41	3
50. Garlic	40	3

ILLUSTRATION V Cont.

	Occurrences	Acceptability
51. Melon	40	3
52. Mushroom	40	3
53. Crab	38	3
54. Fish, misc. small	38	2
55. Lemon	38	3
56. Lizard	38	3
57. Sesame	37	2
58. Guinea fowl	36	2
59. Tamarind	36	2
60. Bambara groundnut	35	1
61. Fig	35	2
62. Antelope	33	1
63. Grape	33	2
64. Manioc, sweet	33	3
65. Bamboo	32	2
66. Buffalo	32	2
67. Shrimp	32	3
68. Larvae, insect	31	3
69. Limes	29	3
70. Millet	29	3
71. Orange, sweet	29	3
72. Pig, wild	28	2
73. Turnip	28	3
74. Avocado	27	2
75. Chick-pea	26	1
76. Gourd, edible	26	3
77. Locust	26	3
78. Jackfruit	25	3
79. Sorghum	26	2

not surprising, is an interesting example of the tendency of societies to systematize and regularize activities whenever possible.

A general overall impression gained from this study is that man tends to extract from his environment a fairly high percentage of the available food resources. In nearly every case, however, there are some curiously unused or unexploited potential resources. Ignorance and revulsion are the most frequently apparent causes. For example, Western culture virtually forbids eating insects, though they are a potential source of nutrition of great importance. Many non-Western societies have no such inhibitions and consume insects in great quantities. As the population explosion continues it may be impossible to continue to ignore these unexploited food resources. Man seems to be physically able to ingest almost anything that does not ingest him first. Almost anything that *can* be consumed — clay, pot sherds, dried cowhide, feces, each other — is consumed

ILLUSTRATION VI

COMPLEMENTARY FOODS

Rank order list of foods used as condiments, sauces, etc. Foods are
listed here when used as complements to other foods though they
may also be listed under other headings in some cases.

	Occurrences	Acceptability
Chili Pepper (Capsicum)	171	2
* Salt	151	3
Sugar cane (sugar and juice)	62	2
Fish, misc.	57	3
Ginger	54	3
Coconut (grated, cream, etc.)	41	3
Garlic (seasoning only)	40	3
Sesame	38	3
Bees, misc. (honey primarily)	36	1
Palm, misc. (oil primarily)	35	2
Onion (seasoning only)	32	3
Sugar plant	32	2
Pepper, black	30	2
Peanut	22	3
Turmeric	22	3
Coriander	20	3
Cow (beef, milk)	18	3
Cloves	17	3
Soybean (soÿ sauce primarily)	17	3
Cardamon	16	2
Cinnamon	15	2
Lime (fruit)	15	3
Mint	15	2
Tamarind	15	3
Beans, misc.	14	3
Mustard	11	3
Okra (seasoning only)	11	3
Rice (as a condiment)	11	2
Bean, Locust, African	10	3
Grape (leaves and fruit)	10	3
Manioc (juice primarily)	10	3
Nutmeg	10	3
Chicken	9	3
Saffron	8	2
Shrimp	8	3
Squash	8	3

*Note: Salt appears to have often been ignored in field reports, consequently this figure is
probably low.

ILLUSTRATION VII

FOOD SOURCES TABOOED

Arranged in rank order by number of groups with any type of taboos.

1. Animals, wild, misc.	114	
Monkeys, misc.	47	
Turtles, misc.	45	
Snakes, misc.	25	
Deer, misc.	22	
Peccary	16	
Pig, wild	16	
Lizards, misc.	12	
Tapir	12	
Armadillo	11	
Frogs, misc.	10	
Leopard	10	415
Rat	9	
Antelope	7	
Hippopotamus	7	
Crabs	6	
Elephant, African	6	
Elephant, Asiatic	2	
Flying Fox	6	
Hyena	6	
Paca	6	
Agouti	5	
Crocodile	5	
Porcupine	5	
Squirrel	5	
2. Animal, domestic, misc.	7	
Chicken, domestic (eggs and meat)	75	
Pig, domestic	70	
Cow, domestic (milk and meat)	58	
Dog	29	
Goat	29	
Sheep	27	345
Duck	12	
Cow, Zebu	12	
Cow, Zebu, female	9	
Cat, domestic	9	
Horse	5	
Ass	3	

ILLUSTRATION VII Cont.

3. Plants, wild and domestic, misc.	88	
Palms, misc.	25	
Rice	25	
Taro	16	
Maize	15	
Coconut	14	
Banana	13	
Sugar cane	9	
Beans, misc.	7	
Mushroom	7	
Breadfruit	6	
Manioc (both)	6	
Squash	6	
Tomato	6	
Potato, sweet	5	258
Millet	5	
Peanut	5	
4. Fish, misc.	86	
Shark	11	
Eel	7	115
Bonito	6	
Catfish	5	
5. Birds, wild, misc.	51	
Pigeon	7	
Vulture	6	69
Rhea	5	
6. Other		
Bee, neuter	17	
Insects, misc.	15	44
Larvae, misc.	6	
Salt	6	

routinely somewhere by some group. Food is what you find, and man is the most adaptable animal of all in this respect.

As a somewhat lighter concluding note, let us imagine that you wished to invite the entire populations of East, South, and Southeast Asia, the Middle East, Africa, Latin America, and Oceania to dinner. What to serve that will be acceptable to nearly all and be reasonably balanced nutritionally This is the menu: chicken, rice, squash, and chili sauce, with tea for a beverage and a banana for desert. Hardly a menu to delight a gourmet, but to most of the world it would be highly acceptable. At all costs avoid serving hippopotamus. Nobody loves a hippopotamus — at least not for dinner.

BIBLIOGRAPHY

This bibliography contains mostly general and survey sources. The specific primary sources which were used for the individual societies studied have not been listed.

Sub-Saharan Africa

Murdock, George Peter. *Africa: Its Peoples and Their Culture History.* New York, McGraw-Hill. 1959.

Hance, William S. *A Geography of Modern Africa.* New York, Columbia University Press. 1964.

Herskovits, Melville J. *The Human Factor in Changing Africa.* New York, Alfred A. Knopf. 1962.

Ottenberg, Simon and Phobe. *Cultures and Societies of Africa.* New York, Random House. 1960.

Smith, Prudence, editor. *Africa in Transition.* London, Max Reinhardt. 1958.

Stamp, L. Dudley. *Africa: A Study in Tropical Development.* New York, John Wiley. 1953.

Middle East

Coon, Carleton S. *Caravan.* New York, Henry Holt. 1951.

Fisher, Sydney Nettleton, Ed. *Social Forces in the Middle East.* Ithaca, New York, Cornell University Press. 1955.

Fisher, W. B. *The Middle East, A Physical, Social and Regional Geography.* London, Methuen. 1950.

Murdock, G. P. *Africa, Its People and Their Culture History.* New York, McGraw-Hill. 1959.

Royal Institute of International Affairs. *The Middle East: A Political and Functional Survey.* 2d ed. London and New York, Royal Institute of International Affairs. 1954.

United Nations. *Review of Economic Conditions in the Middle East.* New York, United Nations. 1952.

Indian Subcontinent

Desai, A. R. *Introduction to Rural Sociology in India.* Bombay, Vora. 1954.

Elwin, Verrier. *The Aboriginals.* Oxford Pamphlets on Indian Affairs, No. 14, Bombay, Oxford University Press, Indian Branch. 1943.

Gilbert, William H. Jr. *Peoples of India.* Smithsonian Institution War Background Studies, No. 18, Washington, Smithsonian Institution. 1944.

Majumdar, D. N. *The Races and Cultures of India.* Allahabad, Kitabistan. 1944.

Brown, Norman W., ed. *India, Pakistan, Ceylon.* Ithaca, Cornell University Press. 1951.

Spate, O. H. K. *India and Pakistan, A General and Regional Geography.* London, Methuen; New York; E. P. Dutton. 1954.

East Asia

Reischauer, Edwin O. and John K. Fairbank. *East Asia: The Great Tradition.* Boston, Houghton Mifflin. 1958.

Cressy, George B. *Asia's Lands and Peoples.* New York, McGraw Hill. 1951.

Wickizer, V. D. and M. K. Bennet. *The Rice Economy of Monsoon Asia.* Stanford University, Food Research Institute. 1941.

Toa Minzoku Meii (Japanese Dictionary of Ethnic Groups in East Asia), Tokyo, Teigoku gakushi In. 1943.

Southeast Asia

Ginsburg, Norton, ed. *The Pattern of Asia.* Englewood Cliffs, N.J., Prentice-Hall. 1958, pp. 290-320, 391-457.

Dobby, E. H. G. *Southeast Asia.* New York, John Wiley. 1950.

Thayer, Philip, W., ed. *Southeast Asia in the Coming World.* Baltimore, Johns Hopkins Press. 1953.

LeBar, Frank M., et al. *Ethnic Groups of Mainland Southeast Asia.* New Haven, Human Relations Area Files. 1964.

Austral-Oceania

General

Keesing, Felix M. *The South Seas in the Modern World*. Rev. ed. New York, John Day. 1945.

Oliver, Douglas L. *The Pacific Islands*. Cambridge, Harvard University Press. 1951.

Robson, R. W. *The Pacific Islands Handbook 1944* (North American Edition). New York, Macmillan. 1945.

Taylor, C. R. H. *A Pacific Bibliography*. Wellington, New Zealand, Polynesian Society. 1951.

Polynesia

Buck, Peter H. *An Introduction to Polynesian Anthropology*. Bernice P. Bishop Museum Bulletin 187, Hawaii. 1945.

Keesing, Felix M. *Social Anthropology in Polynesia*. London, Oxford University Press. 1953.

Melanesia

Elkin, A. P. *Social Anthropology in Melanesia. A Review of Research*. London, Oxford University Press. 1953.

Australia

Elkin, A. P. *The Australian Aborigines*. Garden City, New York, Doubleday Anchor Book N37. 1964.

Greenway, John *Bibliography of the Australian Aborigines and the Native Peoples of Torres Straits to 1959*. Sydney, Angus and Robertson. 1963.

South and Middle America

Steward, Julian H., ed. *Handbook of South American Indians*. 7 vols. Washington, D.C., Bulletin 143 of the Bureau of American Ethnology, Smithsonian Institution. 1946-59.

Steward, Julian H. and Louis C. Faron. *Native Peoples of South America*. New York, McGraw-Hill. 1959.

Wolf, Eric R. *Sons of the Shaking Earth*. Chicago, University of Chicago Press. 1959. (for Mexico and Guatemala)

Rubin, Vera, ed. *Caribbean Studies: A Symposium*. Seattle, University of Washington Press. 1960.

AMERICAN CULTURE AND FOOD HABITS

Communicating through Food in the U.S.A.

NORGE W. JEROME, Ph.D.
Assistant Professor of Nutrition
Department of Preventive Medicine and Community Health
University of Kansas Medical Center
Kansas City, Kansas

Previous speakers have referred to the multiple forces influencing man's use of food. We have learned that food is an integral part of the manifold dimensions in man's life — the biological, cultural, ecological, psychological and social. While exposition of the social and cultural forces operating in exotic cultures arouses our interest and engages our attention, a similar treatment of the multiple forces operating in our native culture tends to confound and frustrate us. The basic reason for this, of course, derives from the very nature of culture itself. This design for living (culture) is so complex and diffusive and we are so influenced by it that it becomes very difficult to step out of it, figuratively, and analyze it objectively.

However, basic understanding of our native cultures, though fraught with frustration, has proved to be very rewarding to those who wish to influence others. For this reason, I have attempted to dissect and analyze American (U.S.) culture and present some basic cultural themes in American society that are expressed in the food habits. Though tentative, the proposition is both challenging and provoking, and I consider myself bold to put it before you for your consideration, discussion, revision, expansion, and hopefully, application. At best, you will have an opportunity for self-analysis and for the modification of current approaches to nutrition education and food distribution.

People communicate who they are as cultural and subcultural groups by the way they use food, since food is but one small facet of the material aspects of our culture. The cultural definitions imply that, for Americans, a set of dietary assumptions, expectations and methods of preparation and service have become integrated into the complex beliefs and practices. Contemporary American culture represents man's highest achievement in technological use of food, i.e. through agricultural and food technology: its diverse forms of application; equipment used in food manufacturing plants; food preservation and transportation machinery; and appliances for preserving, preparing and serving food in the home, in institutional settings, hotels, restaurants, and other food catering establishments.

Food use, as culturally defined at present, depicts at least seven basic "cultural themes" in contemporary American society. Cultural themes are assumptions, beliefs and ideologies (verbalized or non-verbalized) demonstrated by people in the culture and recognized in their art, literature, technologies, dress, housing, food and social institutions. Tentatively, I have identified the cultural themes as: Individualism, Democracy, Capitalism, Industrialism, Pluralism, Youthfulness, and Leisure.

My thesis is that Americans express their Americanism in very specific ways based on their ideologies. Food use represents one way of expressing these ideologies and may be categorized into the seven cultural themes that I have identified. As we analyze these themes, you will note how each one is expressed by individuals or societal institutions in the culture, and through food habits. Each theme, though derived from the philosophies and practices of an earlier era, is currently expressed via the tools, techniques, media and institutions of today. In other words, American culture, which includes its food habits, must be viewed within the setting and framework of the current cybertechnological era. Let us now examine each of the seven themes.

1. *INDIVIDUALISM* — denotes practices based on the assumption that the individual and not society is the paramount consideration or end. Specifically, it refers to individual initiative, interests and action, the myth of the self-made man, and the concept of achievement solely through individual effort. The following statements, familiar to you, depict the self-made man image: "*He* pulled

himself up by *his own* boot straps"; "A self-made man"; "*I* put *myself* through school"; a parent to an 18-year-old: "I gave you a start, now you can make it on your own." The theme of autonomy, self-reliance and self-expression is communicated and demonstrated through self-fulfillment, romantic love, independence, achievement, expenditure of time, energy and money on one's inclinations and desires, and social and geographic mobility.

This particular theme is also communicated through food habits. Some characteristics of individualism in the foodways are autonomy in food selection and consumption; self-expression and ego-gratification through the selection of "image foods," e.g. food items symbolizing reward, reassurance, nostalgia, warmth, comfort, protection, power, strength. The following are some examples of foods selected by individuals to express themselves, communicate emotional states, and define who they are or wish to portray at a given time: "finger foods" — sweet, semi-sweet or salt or semi-salt food items generally referred to as snacks and used as reward and comfort items; soups, milk, and ice cream to express nostalgia and indicate a need for protection and security; thick juicy steaks, caviar and gourmet foods to symbolize achievement or aspirations of success and power.

This partially explains the difficulties encountered by many of you who try to advise people on the proper use of food for therapeutic and preventive measures. Essentially we are asking people to forsake their independence and autonomy and assume a state of dependency contrary to their usual daily routine.

2. *DEMOCRACY* — This general belief in the doctrine of social equality permeates American life and thought, and, like the theme of individualism, rationalizes free expression and choice, individual initiative, and access to knowledge, educational facilities, and other institutional products.

It is important to note that themes and practices that are in conflict with each other modify the outcome of any given cultural theme. In regard to food use, while scientific findings regarding food composition and use are generally available to everyone, other forces in the society permit some people more ready access to these findings than others. In addition, freedom of choice permits the acceptance, rejection, modification or variation in the use of the available scientific information.

While there is, then, general agreement on the relation of food nutrients to health, (often expressed in such terms as "food is good for you"; "food makes you healthy"; "it makes you strong"), self-expression, freedom of choice, independence, the availability of food or food distribution practices at the same time militate against its total expression in food consumption methods and practices. Therefore, despite acceptance of basic nutrition principles garnered from formal and informal education circles, Americans express democratic principles — usually subconsciously — through autonomy in food production, purchasing, selection, preparation and consumption, sometimes with little regard to age, physiological condition, professional advice or the agricultural economy. (The unpopularity of commodity foods, food stamps, and ready-made food budgets probably stems from people's inability to express free choice and demonstrate independence.)

3. *CAPITALISM* — refers to an economic system by which the production, distribution, and exchange of goods is effected by private enterprise and control, under competitive conditions. This statement succinctly describes the American economic system and underlies the food marketing techniques of contemporary American economy. Competition in the marketplace and image building by rival firms account for the numerous varieties of any one food item now available to consumers.

In conformance with the highly developed technological era, marketing techniques stimulate demands, initiate wants and, circularly, respond on demand to those needs and wants initially contrived. The multi-billion dollar food industry, one of the largest civilian consumer industries in the country, is programmed to meet people's biological, psychological and social needs, as well as their "contrived demands." Therefore, food consumption practices are related not only to an individual's biological and psychological needs but also to the needs of investors, manufacturers, and merchandisers — a reality in contemporary American culture. Accordingly, these external factors operating in the marketplace are communicated via food habits. People buy the "new improved" brands as well as lower price tags — they infrequently purchase food as a source of nutrients.

4. *PLURALISM* — The presence of different ethnic, racial, socio-economic and age-graded groups is peculiar to American society. The country's history and its method of settling, growth, and devel-

opment essentially define the particulars as well as the peculiar nature of the American pluralistic society. Individuals and groups, depending upon race, ethnicity and socio-economic status, form different stratas linearly, and varieties of pockets horizontally.

These realities find expression in the foodways of the people. Pluralism, as defined, is communicated through inequities in the distribution of food, qualitatively as well as quantitatively. Unequal food distribution or social distinctions in food consumption patterns are again interconnected with the cultural themes discussed previously — an example of the integrated and pervasive nature of culture.

The presence of various subcultural groups (ethnic, regional, racial) in the culture is expressed through wide variations in food consumption practices, and traditionalism and non-traditionalism in the foodways. There appears to be a hierarchy of dietary habits in American culture. 1) There are the *primary food habits* that are generally described by outsiders as American. They transcend class, regional, age-related and subcultural eating habits and include food items, mode of cooking, aroma, seasoning ingredients, eating environment and cooking and serving utensils. Examples of food items which, when incrporated into a specific climate or environment, determine Americanism in the food habits are hamburgers, ground meat, beef, chicken, sliced white wheat bread (toasted or untoasted), buns, wieners, luncheon meats, fruit drinks, juice and carbonated beverages, apples, white potatoes, apple pie, milk, ice cream, and coffee.

2) *The secondary food habits* equivalent to the basic eating patterns of particular subgroups in the American society are peculiar to social class, subculture and region, and are related to the specific life-style of a people. They characterize the adjustments, solutions and compromises made by people to the requisites of everyday life. The basic eating pattern of specific subgroups essentially underscore traditionalism in the foodways — Pennsylvania Dutch, Polish, Ozarks, New England, Southern.

3) An *accessory eating pattern* obtains in the culture and may be defined as the incorporation of non-traditional food items or entire meals into the total foodways, thus underscoring non-traditionalism, acculturation, assimilation, and eclecticism, and communicating extant variety of dietary practices in the total American culture.

5. *INDUSTRIALISM* — The predominant theme and influential force in mid-twentieth century American life is communicated

through food habits. This theme is expressed by the mass production of goods resulting from the application of basic science to agricultural, food and industrial technology. Some characteristics of its effect on society and societal institutions are as follows:

a. Reduction in manpower needed for primary food production. (Only a minority of 7-8 percent of the population produces food.)

b. Availability of large amounts and varieties of foods.

c. Entry of the traditional "home food processor" to the civilian labor force. (One worker in three is a woman; women and girls sixteen years of age and over accounted for two-thirds of the increase in the civilian labor force during 1963-1968. The forecast is for 30 million in 1970.)

d. Use of organized manpower for commercial food processing and service.

e. Large-scale food production, processing and preparation in manufacturing plants.

The effect of this twentieth-century phenomenon on food consumption practices is well known to all of us. The culture theme is expressed in the primary and secondary food habits and the accessory eating patterns of Americans. The prevalence of a variety of raw, processed, and prepared foods throughout the year communicates the richness and abundance of the harvest.

Food purchasing is the major form of "food production" in an industrialized society; this phenomenon needs no documentation to members of the society that introduced the world to the supermarket. Potatoes, tomatoes, lettuce, carrots and onions are "gathered" in cellophane bags and/or small cardboard boxes; apples and berries are "gathered" in bushel baskets. Romaine, head and leaf lettuce "grow" side by side in the produce section of the supermarket; in one "garden" the size of a master bedroom, on any morning, afternoon or evening, one may "gather" peaches, nectarines, grapes, cherries, apricots, strawberries, blueberries, asparagus, egg plant, turnips, cabbage, squash, tomatoes, celery, carrots, cantaloupes, onions, radishes, corn, green pepper, potatoes, beans, broccoli or cucumber, depending upon his inclination and "gathering" or purchasing ability.

In "gathering" fruits and vegetables one may have the awesome task of trying to select one of four or five varieties of a particular product.

A few steps from the vegetable orchard-garden one could select one of fifty-two meat products vacuum packed in plastic film. Competing with each other for the consumer's attention as he walks in a trance from aisle to aisle are fish, poultry, and meat of many varieties, descriptions and cuts; cereals, condiments, fruit drinks, fruit juices and carbonated beverages — all appealing to the eye and convenient to use (although their nutrient content has been long lost during processing or on the assembly line). Often, instead of selecting foods, Mrs. Consumer chooses brilliant colors, package designs and displays. She collects formulated, health enriched, defatted, artificially sweetened, simulated, fortified and weakened foods. Mrs. Consumer is forced to make a selection — why she is not sure. In her trance she often forgets to read the small print that sometimes describes the ingredients that have been added to her meal, beverage or food.

6. *LEISURE* — deals with hours and ways of behavior in which one is free to be himself. As a cultural theme, leisure is inextricably bound with the themes already discussed. Cultural forces have acted and interacted in such a manner that a good deal of free time is now available to most people, and many are in a position to take advantage of leisure through recreation, entertainment, hobbies, education and travel. Diners, restaurants, cafeterias and snack stands — all associated with leisure — have sprung up in answer to this new demand.

Food merchandisers have also responded to the current use of time by marketing a wide variety of "finger" foods and snack items associated with leisure. Also it is evident that they initiated or at least catalyzed current trends by providing food items and meals that require a minimum of time in preparation. They have also cooperated by packaging foreign dishes, delicacies and gourmet food items that are generally associated with leisure hours, vacations and travel. Consumption by Americans of these relatively new lines of food expresses use of time, frequency of eating and the textural quality and size of leisure-time foods. (It is important to note that popular snack foods are crisp and crunchy and come in bite-sized pieces.)

7. *YOUTHFULNESS* — That youth and youthful figures are deified in American society is probably an understatement. Beauty, vigor and vitality are sold and encouraged in most areas of daily life including food consumption or lack thereof. Food and nutrient (vitamins) consumption, especially the consumption of formulated foods and the abstention from "fattening" foods are designed for the retention or recapture of youth and vitality. In many instances, food selection is based on caloric content — often erroneously — and a state or quality of lightness perceived by many to be associated with reducing poundage or fostering youth. Dry toast, cottage cheese, black coffee, "diet pop" and certain vegetable juices fall in this category. Thus stems the popularity of "health" foods, sexy cookbooks and beverage potions that promise eternal youth and everlasting vitality.

Essentially, food habits represent the nature and character of U.S. society and underscore such intangibles as value systems, beliefs, expectations, desires, aspirations, social status and prestige symbols, as well as such measurable factors as social and cultural pluralism, economic status, and level of technological development.

Americans communicate who they are by their food habits. By looking at *what* people eat, *how, where, when, how much* and *how often,* one notes expressions of ideologies applicable to Individualism, Democracy, Capitalism, Pluralism, Industrialism, Leisure and Youthfulness. However, these themes are not discrete and separate; neither are they cohesive and coherent. Continuities, conflicts, idosyncrasies, discord and inconsistencies abound. The concerned practitioner should be alert to the myriad ways in which culture is manifested in order to utilize meaningful educational approaches and appropriate corrective measures to programs, issues and events. Measures that are not appropriate to given situations will prove not only inconsequential but utterly futile in terms of attaining a particular goal.

Specifically, with regard to food, Americans wish to express their independence, affluence, other-directedness, social class, youthfulness, ethnicity or subcultural group membership. This is what it means to be an American in terms of food use and behavior.

The following chart will summarize American themes of expression in food habits:

SELECTED THEMES IN AMERICAN CULTURE EXPRESSED IN FOOD HABITS

Theme	Theme Expression by Individuals, Society or Societal Institutions	Theme Communication Through Food Habits
Individualism	Self-fulfillment Educational achievement Romantic love Social and geographic mobility Success through individual effort Independence Freedom to expend time, energy and money on individual inclination	Autonomy in food selection and consumption Self-gratification by selecting "image foods," e.g. food items symbolizing ego-gratification—success, warmth, security, comfort, reward, love, reassurance, power, strength Personality expression through food selection and consumption
Democracy	Freedom of choice Access to formal and informal education	Autonomy in food production, purchasing, selection, preparation and consumption with little regard to age, physiological condition or professional advice Food use relating food nutrients to health
Capitalism	Competitive merchandising in the distribution of goods Image building of brand names	Food purchasing and consumption based on merchandising techniques, contrived demands and brand image

Theme	Theme Expression by Individuals, Society or Societal Institutions	Theme Communication Through Food Habits
Industrialism	Application of basic science to agricultural, food and industrial technology	Prevalence of a variety of raw, processed, and prepared foods throughout the year
	Reduction in manpower needed for primary food production	Food purchasing
	Availability of large amounts and varieties of food	Food preparation and consumption away from home
	Entry of the traditional home food processor to civilian labor force	Consumption of a variety of enriched, fortified and formulated foods and beverages
	Use of organized manpower for commercial food processing and service	Consumption of "health" foods
	Large scale food production, processing and preparation in manufacturing plants	
Leisure	Expenditures on recreation, entertainment, hobbies, education, travel	Consumption of food away from home
		Consumption of wide variety of "snack," leisure-time or "finger" foods
	Marketing of hundreds of "finger" and "snack" foods	Consumption of gourmet foods & packaged foreign dishes

Theme	Theme Expression by Individuals, Society or Societal Institutions	Theme Communication Through Food Habits
Pluralism	Presence of different ethnic, racial, socio-economic and age-graded groups	Unequal distribution of foods Social distinction in food consumption patterns Variations in food consumption practices Traditionalism and non-traditionalism in food ways Primary food habits associated with American culture. Secondary food habits associated with social class, ethnic & cultural background Accessory eating pattern related to exposure to a variety of food consumption practices
Youthfulness	Statements, claims and beliefs concerning food as aids to beauty, vigor and vitality	Food and nutrient consumption or abstinence to retain or recapture youth and vitality Wide consumption of low-calorie food and beverages

SELECTED REFERENCES

American Women 1963-1968. Report of the Interdepartmental Committee on the Status of Women. Washington, D.C. 1968.

Galbraith, John N. *The Affluent Society.* Boston: Houghton-Mifflin. 1958.

Kaplan, Max. *Leisure in America.* New York: John Wiley & Sons. 1960.

Packard, Vance. *The Hidden Persuaders.* New York: David McKay. 1957.

Taeuber, K. E., et al. *Migration in the United States.* Public Health Monograph No. 77, U. S. Department of Health, Education and Welfare. 1968.

DISCUSSION

QUESTIONS TO DR. MOORE AND DR. JEROME

DR. THEODORATUS: I would like to add one comment in regard to the factor that Professor Jerome mentioned about affluence, and I speak as an anthropologist. I started in archeology, and archeologists are primarily concerned with refuse, in essence what is left in the garbage dumps of civilizations. What goes into people's garbage cans, things that they purchase which they are literally forced to by the advertising media, whether these are cereals that the children buy which they will never eat (no one could stand to eat it, at least this is an adult's point of view), this other sort of massive data for symbolism in regard to food habits should be examined. I am not sure if Dr. Jerome would make a comment on that or not.

DR. JEROME: I remember once commenting on the richness of the urine of Americans in general. I think it relates to the same thing. What you throw away you need not simply put in your garbage pail or your garbage disposal. But also you can dispose of it in your bathroom, and I think that for the most part many people do so.

QUESTION: In view of these situations, should we worry more about nutrition education or food supplementation?

ANSWER: (Dr. Jerome) The reason I was trying to pass the buck is that I do not give advice. I say as the catalyst, the devil's advocate, I don't know answers, and so I can't tell you what you should worry about, but I will state that I believe that our approach to education is not entirely appropriate. We nutrition educators and dietitians, I don't know that we are the influencing force in terms of nutrition education. Somehow I believe that we will have to change our approach and educate the people who are motivating and influencing people in their food consumption. I would also recommend consumer education, like teaching nutrition in the grocery store, or probably food supplementation, because this is where it is.

ANSWER: (Dr. Moore) One of the things that struck me, I think I mentioned it during the course of the study that I described earlier, is the tremendous range of diets that people are able to subsist on and get along very well. This makes me always a little doubtful when I see some sort of ideal diet or *the* diet that is prescribed as being the thing people ought to eat. I am pretty well convinced that people can get along on almost anything. This may not be the best possible diet from the point of view of warding off disease, maintaining perfect health and muscle tone, but it is pretty obvious to me that there is a tremendous range of diets that serve the purpose of keeping people going.

QUESTION: Dr. Schaefer, will you say something about that?

DR. SCHAEFER: In a way, I take issue because if one looks at mortality data in the developing countries, he will find that certainly people in societies have survived. I hope that concerning the health aspects, however, we are not going to be satisfied with just sheer survival. I can't argue with you. In fact, the Indians on the continent of India have survived, and in Pakistan the people have survived. However, when one realizes that the cumulative mortality rate is something like 50 percent dead by age seventeen, one realizes this is interwoven between nutrition, infectious disease, and many other ecological factors. I think it is interesting to recall that this is the same stage we were at in the United States in 1908. We had a mortality index of 50 percent dead by age twenty-one. This happened to be the first time we took a census and tried to calculate this sort of statement.

I believe in a way what you said is true. People can eat a wide variety of foods and most of the world subsists on the cereal type commodity supplemented with legumes. The three cereals are obvious; first there is rice, then wheat, and then corn. But you cannot have children survive on just wheat, rice or corn. Again, in the United States I think we are looking for answers now as to whether we can educate the population on getting the right mix of foods. I like the suggestion that perhaps we have been looking at the wrong places to educate them. Perhaps the best place is through the grocery stores, the people who are really doing the selling job; hopefully we can get them to become less commodity oriented and more nutrition oriented. I don't really know whether that is possible, but I would surely like to try it.

QUESTION: It would occur to me from these cultural themes that one might see how people could communicate through devices other than food, an approach to changing food habits. In other words, an attempt to play on one's individualism. Are there mechanisms other than food that could be used in a different mix? Maybe an approach to changing food habits might be an approach by looking at other avenues for expression. Would this seem reasonable?

ANSWER: (Dr. Jerome) It seems reasonable, and I think that this is what I had in mind when I developed these themes, because food is one way, as I suggested, by which you express these various idealogies. I think it is about time that we revised our approaches and this method of communicating with people; the way they themselves communicate is appealing to me. I would like to follow through on this sometime in terms of developing demonstration programs to test this.

QUESTION: I would like to ask both of you, where do you think food, diet, and the patterns of eating are going in the United States, say in the next ten years? Would you like to stick your neck out on this?

ANSWER: (Dr. Moore) Well, it is pretty obvious, getting back to what we were talking about before, that pre-packaged foods are going to be more and more dominant. The housewife doesn't seem to want to be bothered with fresh vegetables, etc., anymore. Everything is going to be packaged. You see it more everytime you go into the supermarket. What it is going to be like ten years from now I would not hazard to guess, but I will say one thing. I think it will be increasingly hard to buy anything fresh in an ordinary supermarket.

ANSWER: (Dr. Jerome) I am afraid I left my crystal ball at home, however I will make this comment. I did a study in Milwaukee using the participant observation approach. I stayed in the community for seven months and really learned in depth how people ate. These were blacks who were born in the South and migrated to an urban situation. You know collard greens supported the Southern way of eating, greens of various forms. In many instances, I won't go into all the details, I identifed different groups, I believe, in these hierarchies, and I found a group that I believed to be the most aculturated of the total sample. These people did not consume fresh greens. They consumed frozen greens for the most part.

The interesting point I want to make here is that with the change in the use of the common food that was packaged and preserved differently, there came about a conservation of nutrients, because no longer did the people cook the greens for a long period of time with ham hocks, etc. They were using a new product, so to speak, so they followed the package directions. You cook them for five to eight minutes with a little spread or bacon. Consequently, I don't know that the trend that I see of everything being packaged is going to be all bad if one is looking specifically at conservation of nutrients.

It is important that we all watch what is happening and not discourage people from doing what comes to them naturally because we have a good deal of professional background or know-how. People live, and they must live, in their way; they devise methods, somehow, to survive. I thought this observation was particularly important (I haven't published it any place other than in my thesis): the use of frozen vegetables, the preparation of frozen vegetables in a manner different from the traditional, and in a manner that would please the host of nutritionists and dietians, warmed my heart.

DR. MOORE: There is one other thing about the advent of more frozen and pre-packaged vegetables and food stuffs of one kind or another. I think there is probably going to be a trend to a greater variety available in these things. For instance, I noticed this past winter that one of the local supermarkets in New Haven was featuring frozen Jerusalem artichokes. Now I am not all that thrilled with Jerusalem artichokes, but I think perhaps this is the trend. Who knows? We may have caro and whatnot in the supermarket before long.

QUESTION: Having spent a big part of my working career in nutrition working with poverty groups, I can't help commenting when you talk of education and cultural patterns as being big influences. Just talking about these two factors is not enough if we are going to attack the problem when we know there is a minimum income under which it is difficult, to say the least, if not impossible, to have an adequate diet. I throw this open for rejection or whatever you want. It doesn't make sense to talk about education programs in nutrition without talking about an adequate income with which to educate them from.

ANSWER: (Dr. Jerome) I touched on this in some of my themes, if you will recall, in terms of food distribution. People *do* purchase foods right now, even if they spend only a dollar a day, even if their income is $30.00 per week; they purchase foods! Shouldn't we approach the thing from an educational standpoint? They are buying the things that are there.

RESPONSE: My point is I think we are missing the boat if we don't approach the problem at the root cause, and the whole problem instead of many fragmented parts as we are doing.

DR. JEROME: Meaning going to Washington, getting the people jobs, this sort of thing?

RESPONSE: No, I mean everybody and his brother going out and educating people about nutrition.

CHAIRMAN: I think you are talking at cross purposes. She is being facetious in terms of talking about everybody and his brother educating. I think what she basically means is the income problem. She is talking about going to Washington and getting jobs.

ANSWER: (Dr. Jerome) I did not want to bring up my pet theme at this particular time, but friends of mine know that this I perceive as one method of attack. I don't believe that I have appropriate data on hand right now to verbalize on it at this time.

ANSWER: (Dr. Schaefer) Along these lines, it has certainly been brought out today that adequate income certainly does not insure adequate diet. There are many extremely badly nourished people who have all the money in the world. Obviously we can get down to the nitty-gritty of what is wrong with the whole society, but I think we are talking here about what we can do about nutrition.

QUESTION: Dr. Jerome, I was wondering, in looking at your seven themes as discreetly as you can, which do you think will be the most susceptible to developing famines, and which would persist the longest? In other words, if things were tough and the food supply became limited, which would fold first and which would survive the longest?

ANSWER: (Dr. Jerome) Individualism would survive the longest, I believe. But I said that they were intertwined. If you have nothing but garbage to eat, you will eat the piece of garbage that appeals to you the most.

COMMENT: I always have to get on the other side of the table when we are talking about poverty and those nutrition problems which do exist, and plenty of people are concerned about them. But the problem in the U.S., in totality, is not poverty; it is obesity. In this case we do need some new way to help people learn how to manage their food.

DR. JEROME: Would you suggest, Dr. Dupont, that we use the same methods as used by the motivators?

DR. DUPONT: If anybody could teach us how to motivate, I would be ready to do it. This the problem. I don't know, and we have to think of new ways.

DR. JEROME: But there are ways. Our food habits have changed. The question is, looking at the same things I said, what are the influential factors?

DR. DUPONT: In spite of the fact that youthfulness is so wonderful, we are still suffering, in twenty or twenty-five percent of the people, with gross obesity.

DR. JEROME: I believe that we may have to resort to the same methods used by the motivators in the society, merchandisers, etc. If you are looking at a crash program, I don't know of any other way, but it is a very expensive way.

V

DIMENSIONS TODAY
AND TOMORROW

FINDINGS AND IMPLICATIONS OF THE
NATIONAL NUTRITION SURVEY

ARNOLD E. SCHAEFER, Ph.D.
Chief, Nutrition Program
Regional Medical Programs Service
Department of Health, Education and Welfare
Bethesda, Maryland

Introduction

The goal of the National Nutrition Survey is to have examined in the United States approximately 70,000 individuals by the first of 1970. Our survey is composed of a medical clinical examination of every individual who is selected to participate. This individual is a member of a family selected on a random basis. Individuals receive complete physical examinations. In many states parameters other than nutrition are studied. Depending upon the capability or interest of each state, this can include examination for parasites, eye and hearing tests, and special biochemical studies such as serum lipids and trace minerals. A blood and a urine sample is taken from each individual and these are analyzed for some of the key nutrients. In addition, approximately one-half of the total population receives an individual dietary recall. We are also obtaining a large battery of data on the social and economic status of all families.

We had several objectives, some political, some to give us answers which would either confirm or disagree with our previous data. By disagreeing I mean possessing the cold facts to convince Congress that 1) either the current programs directed toward the poverty groups are effective or 2) that they are not effective. Specifically, is the current food commodity distribution program having any impact on improving the health of the people who are receiving it?

Is the current food stamp plan effective under its current aegis in improving health? We are not interested in the economic aspect, but we have been and are convinced that nutrition is a health problem.

I have been accused of being anti-agricultural. I came from the schools of agriculture and I worked in them. I am sympathetic to agriculture and I appreciate, I am sure, as well as anyone that the United States is a land of food surplus. We have the most sophisticated food producing capability in the world. We are supposed to have one of the best education systems in the world. With these two advantages plus good health, there is no reason why we should tolerate any degree of malnutrition. I know this is a high goal. If I have had one chip on my shoulder during my fifteen yeras of government service it has been due to the fact that the Public Health Service and HEW have given only lip service to nutrition. There has been a complete lack of an appreciation that nutrition is an integral part of preventive medicine.

In our affluent society, people neglect to see some of the problems of the less fortunate members of our society. Our efforts are directed toward medical care and treatment. I am not against that. As far as I am concerned, however, nutrition is preventive medicine, and I want to do all I can to see that we stand on that premise. Prevention of malnutrition starts with the pregnant mother and pre-school child. By the time the "fat-age" group is reached, the problem is nearly controlled. This is the theme upon which I would like to see an ongoing nutrition program build. The $64 question is, "Do we have severe problems of malnutrition in the United States?"

The National Nutrition Survey

Our current data is based on a preselected 10 states from a geographic distribution that we hoped would include population groups in ghetto areas, the rural poor, and migrant workers, and would take into consideration some of the environmental variations within the U.S. These states are Texas, Louisiana, West Virginia, Kentucky, South Carolina, Massachusetts, New York, Michigan, Washington, and California. Under this arrangement, an obvious void appears in the midwest. This gap was left on the assumption that we would have funds to enable us to do an extensive study on the Indian reservations and to select two or three different states in the Great

Plains area. We are still hoping for them. The first year of operation we received no funds to do anything for the Indian reservations. We did manage to beg and borrow enough to do a small study on the Navajo Indian Reservation which was supported primarily by the Department of Agriculture.

We have now finished five states. All field activities have been completed in Texas, Louisiana, Kentucky, upstate New York and Michigan. We now have two teams in California and two in the state of Washington. The surveys of New York City and West Virginia have been started. The funds to negotiate the contracts for Massachusetts and South Carolina were not available until 5:00 p.m. on the 30th of June, so there is still much to be done to start those two surveys. It is erroneous to state that we are studying only poverty. Our sample is selected from the lower quartile of income areas identified by the Census Bureau based on the 1960 Census. This means that if our sample is properly selected we should be talking about one-fourth of the population of the United States with distribution between rural, urban, and semi-rural populations.

We are primarily working with poverty groups. We are using the Orshansky Index of Poverty to classify the families or individuals according to the poverty index. This takes into consideration whether the family is rural or urban, size of the family and location of the family as far as cost of living. By using the Orshansky Index we find that 58 to 60 percent of the people are living below the poverty index. That allows approximately $3,000 to $3,300 for a family of four. We do have a spread in income, however, which was set in Texas and has not been changed yet, from $185 per year for a family to $42,000.

Using the Iowa Growth Standard we are finding evidence of growth retardation in preschool children. There are about 10 to 15 percent of children below the 4th percentile. The children 0-6 years of age are retarded approximately from 9 months to 2½ years by the time they are age six. This picture is not much different from what we have seen in some of the developing countries. No one can argue against problems of growth retardation.

Is all this growth retardation due to malnutrition? I am not sure. I am convinced that malnutrition is probably the largest contributing factor. We found, for example, that about 4 to 5 percent of the 0-3 year olds had evidence of rickets. We scientists said it had been eradicated twenty or thirty years ago in the United States. Is it reappearing? Is it due to ignorance? Is it due to changing some of our food marketing and processing procedures? There are a whole battery of nutrients that we can analyze in tissue, and we are saying that tissue levels are so low that if it was your child or mine going to a pediatrician, he would immediately start therapy.

We found 18 cases of Bitot's spots. This looks like a little hunk of beer foam in the white of the eye. These have historically been described as being due to Vitamin A deficiency. I was unaware of any report of a case of Bitot's spots in children in the United States until this survey. We have traced 18 cases out of 28,000 people sampled. We have had 7 cases of flagrant kwashiorkor or marasmus. I would not expect to find *one* in the United States, and I am not ready to buy the fact that there were 7 that had been undetected. Overseas we do not find this many during a survey because these children are either dead or in the hospital.

Again, some of these cases are not necessarily due to the fact that the people do not have sufficient food. It is due to ignorance, and I think much of it can be traced to changes in the food being supplied to the specific population.

It is not enough to say that an individual has an anemia. We are interested in being able to determine what kind of anemia. Is it iron deficiency or folic acid deficiency or a multiple etiology? The U. S. Army Medical Research and Nutrition Laboratory here in Denver is serving as our key laboratory to do all of these analyses. In addition, it is serving as our referee laboratory.

Vitamin A

The Vitamin A picture should draw our attention to the fact that we are undergoing a change in diet. We could be on the brink of experiencing a severe outbreak of Vitamin A deficiency. I again mention the Bitot's spots. We did not see a blind child in our survey. Of course, I think most of you know that any person on a diet low in or void of Vitamin A shows reduced liver stores, tissue stores, and serum levels. In our international work, if the child or adult has a level of 20 mcg/100 ml of serum, or less, there is a real health risk. I have seen cases of xerophthalmia, severe eye lesions, occur in children at Vitamin A levels of 10 mcg or less. Blindness due to Vitamin A deficiency can be prevented for the cost of a candy bar per year for each child, provided one could find a mechanism for getting Vitamin A into the child's diet. The best food source of Vitamin A has been, and still is, full fat milk.

We were criticized by some of the medical profession who said: "Maybe your standards were wrong and that is why you are having such a high incidence of Vitamin A deficiency." I am just bull-headed enough to say our standards are not wrong. We used them all over the world, where Vitamin A deficient blind children occur not by the tens but by the thousands. I do not want the United States to fall back to that sloppy habit of saying: "Let us wait until we see some blind kids before we get perturbed about the Vitamin A problem."

Some new figures emphasizing this point: Out of over 1,000 pre-school children studies in Alabama, Louisiana, Mississippi, and Tennessee the percentage of children who have less than 20 micrograms of Vitamin A is: 26 in Alabama, 35 in Louisiana, 16 in Mississippi and 94 percent in Tennessee. Mothers had much higher Vitamin A levels, but 5 to 6 percent of the mothers of these children had low Vitamin A levels.

Vitamin C

The Vitamin C problem is a little different: In Louisiana, 18 percent of the children had levels of less than 0.2 mg; in Alabama, 48 percent; 9 percent of the mothers in Louisiana, and 29 percent in Mississippi revealed these low levels.

Vitamin C deficiency is a problem found in all age groups. The prevalence of low blood serum Vitamin C levels in various age groups ranges from 10 to 12 percent to 16 or 18 percent. These data, computed on the basis that serum levels of Vitamin C are less than 0.2 mg/100 ml, again indicate a high risk problem. About 5 percent of the population had levels of less than 0.1 mg. Acknowledging the sensitivity of the methods that we are using, it is at this 0.1 mg level that one expects to see some physical signs of border-line scurvy developing. One of the best correlations we have had in our international studies is the percentage of people who at levels of less than 0.1 mg will start showing evidence of bleeding, puffy, "scorbutic" type gums. We know very well that this gum lesion can be caused by pyorrhea and other things. We have found that 5 percent of the population examined to date had "scorbutic" type gums, 5 had levels of serum Vitamin C or 0.1 mg or less, and a larger percentage had what we term borderline levels.

There is a report on nutrition survey of the Navajos which was conducted in 1954. The findings in 1954 and the findings in 1969 of our survey in Greiswood (Navajo Reservation) are very similar. They still show the same problems. We could not get anyone to litsen in 1954. Jointly with the military, we conducted a survey in the Blackfeet Indian Reservation of Montana in 1961. The findings there were similar to what we are finding today. In 1961 nobody listeend. The study was made and the report submitted, and that is as far as we got.

Where should we go from here? What are the possibilities? What, as nutrition scientists, can we do? How can we stimulate federal bureaucracy; stimulate people to deliver? What is required to insure adequate nutrition for our population?

Dental Problems

I failed to mention that there are some associated findings that are probably as critical as problems of malnutrition. Over 90 percent of the population studied had a severe dental problem. There was an average of six teeth in need of immediate filling. There was an average of eleven teeth, that is, one out of every three in your mouth, that required filling or pulling. Eighteen percent of the people we studied indicated that it hurt to chew, and that as a result they changed some of their food habits. We found a 12-year old child who was dentureless. The public health branch of dentistry supervised and conducted the dental aspects of our survey. Their appraisal is that they had not seen any worse mouths in any study they had done. This has a relationship to nutrition that we cannot ignore. Welfare allows $25 for dental care. If you have eleven teeth which require filling you know how far $25 goes — if you can find a dentist.

In many of these areas there are no health facilities. This means we must rely on paramedical help if we are going to be sincere in

addressing ourselves to problems in the poverty areas. Medical practitioners are not going to address these problems — they are busy;
they are involved in treatment and not prevention. When one speaks
of the problems in the poverty groups, he is primarily speaking of
people who do not have access to health facilities, or if they do, it
is only under emergencies.

Obesity

Let me go a step further to indicate one of the big problems —
this is obesity. I gave up trying to talk about obesity at the Senate
hearings. I can assure you we are going to talk about it the next time.
Fifty percent of the members that we studied were 20 percent or
more overweight. Many of them were anemic, and had low serum
albumin and Vitamin A levels. Obesity or fatness is due primarily
to the kind of diet. There are other causes of obesity but the primary
one is a higher caloric intake than expenditure. When you realize
that some of the dietary intakes are predominantly high in carbohydrates and low in protein, it is easy to understand why obesity
occurs. It is difficult to reduce somebody on that type of diet. We
have another obesity problem. In one county, if an obese mother
comes for food commodity distribution neither she nor her family
is certified as eligible for food.

Welfare Programs

There are state rules and regulations which determine who is eligible for welfare and who is eligible for food stamps or food commodities. I can see nothing uniform in the administration of these
mandates.

There are 50 contracts for welfare with 50 states. When you get
in the game of food donations and food stamps the rules and regulations must be multiplied by the 3,000 odd counties, because virtually each county has a different set. Less than 10 percent of our
sample population below the poverty index are actually recipients
of either food commodities or food stamps. If you put this on a
dollar basis, the average dollar value per person per day for those
receiving food commodities is about 17 cents. However, this figure
is going to come out closer to 12 cents for the U.S. as a whole. Try
to feed somebody for 12 cents on the food commodity distribution

items; there may be 22 items, but we have not found a family yet who received 22 items. They usually are lucky if they receive 11. In the case of food stamps, the average dollar value per person per day is about 22 cents. Now the Department of Agriculture has indicated that the least cost diet is 75 cents. Secondly, 50 percent of those people who are getting food stamps or food commodities are already on welfare, but they have had to be recertified in most cases. I do not know of anything that reveals more duplication of effort.

I was pleased that in the last testimony by Agriculture and HEW, for the first time in my history, the Secretaries sat at the same bench. Furthermore, they were in agreement. HEW was not interested in taking over the food commodity distribution program or the food stamp program. However, the Secretary is looking forward to the day when food will be considered part and parcel of a uniform welfare payment. Secretary Hardin was sitting next to him saying he wanted to phase out the commodity distribution system as quickly as possible and looked to the day when food stamps would be incorporated as part of the welfare payment. I think this makes sense in the long run, but money alone will not solve the problem. Congress can always talk well, but unless we can be sure that the people in dire need receive aid in the form of instruction on how to buy, and what to buy, the program will be of little use to improve nutritional health.

For the long run and for the immediate short run there are some real needs. A good federal policy guideline that recognizes that nutrition is a part of preventive medicine, and recognizes that the Public Health Service and HEW have never really supported the field, is necessary. I think it ridiculous that the U.S. has not had some sort of surveillance (or monitoring) system to keep abreast of our changing food supply as it relates to the health of the people and the changing migration of people. This can never be effective until it is done at the local level. We are now fighting the battle of the bureaucrats by saying that we do not believe that monitoring should be done through a federal inspection team. It would be more successful to have centers capable of continually monitoring or conducting surveillance on nutritional health status within the states. I would like to see states, towns, or local communities devise ways and means of trying to determine how we can affect the assurance of proper nutrition for all. If we can do it for the lower quartile of income groups, I am convinced it will rub off on the higher echelon. We usually start the other way, educate those who are educated. Now the challenge is educating those who really need help.

Education Programs

I am convinced of two things. First, our procedures or techniques of educating people across the board in good food habits and nutrition are outmoded. Second, there is such an urgent need now that we must take a new approach. I do not know what the exact new approach should be. We pointed out in our testimony to Congress that there are two channels to reach the mother. In the U.S. those channels basically are the school system and the food stores. I doubt whether or not the health centers can serve this purpose, because there are millions of people who never see a health center or who do not have one. How do we put health into the school system or into the food distribution chain to make sure we reach the needy mothers? This is where we need help.

We have talked of selecting several public schools and determine how we can reach the first grader all the way through high school. We should really concentrate on the teenage girl who will be a mother in the next few years and motivate her to proper food habits and nutrition. I think we could show her some slides and some data on the high risk of mental retardation in low birth weight infants. I am not interested in waiting until someone proves to me that in the United States malnutrition can cause mental retardation. We have supported studies in Chile, Guatemala, and Africa in the past ten years and the risk is great. When one has growth retardation in the child, a low birth weight infant, the risk of mental and neurological retardation is there. Many of today's physicians who advise "Do not gain any weight in the last trimester of pregnancy" are potential contributors to this serious problem. This is reaching the ridiculous state. The risk is there. Fifty percent of low birth-weight infants face a real danger of being mentally retarded.

We must get to the teenage girl and not talk simply of the four food groups, but start showing her some of the data. Dr. Beaseley in Louisiana has collected some valuable information on teenage girls. Dr. McGanity, head of obstetrics and gynecology at Texas

University Medical Branch, is going to help us make a film on some of the nutrition problems that come into the clinic in the lower income groups on teenage girls. I think this sort of information, if it could be shown in a class, would be helpful.

I am not saying you must have a course in nutrition. In fact, I doubt that would succeed. Nutrition could be taught in history. An interesting course could be taught in history if Goldberger's experiments on pellagra in the United States or the story of Vitamin C were discussed. Nutrition could be incorporated into mathematics courses. Let students calculate some of the calories or some of the food requirements of their county or state or of the world. Nutrition can and must be incorporated into health courses. I do not mean just sit down, take a deep breath, eat so much milk, eggs and meat. I mean to really stimulate these students as to the physiological function, the utilization of nutrients and what it means as far as they are concerned or their families are concerned. This could work from kindergarten up through high school.

Manpower Needs

We have been through a real battle saying that there is an urgent need to support manpower. Supporting manpower means supporting the training and underwriting the jobs of a battery of nutritionists, be they dietitians, home economists, paramedical specialists, nurses, nutritionists, etc., who can get out, relate to and work with the poverty or welfare programs and the food aides that the Department of Agriculture now has. There are, beyond any doubt, segments of the population which need special consideration. For example, the aging require a sociological approach. Why do the aged quit eating and really change food habits? Is it teeth, lack of interest, lack of knowledge, or the fact that they do not have the resources? Here is a real need for manpower.

We have tried to get funds earmarked to support nutrition training and have gotten nowhere. We have made no progress since over 90 percent of the manpower funds is used to train more physicians. Let me give you an example. There is a need for 7,000 doctors per year. There is assurance that will go through. There is need for a quarter of a million nurses, a shortage right now, yet very little federal money is going to support nursing. Nutrition receives even less support. Last year we identified two new fellowship programs that were supported by NIH. What we really must emphasize is the need for the paramedical personnel that will help by working with the schools, with the communities, with the action programs, and really deliver service. This means getting right to the mother, and it may have to be in the home. I would like to see the day when we teach all teenage girls. Then within 10 to 20 years all mothers perhaps would be educated and would appreciate the problems of malnutrition.

How do we take care of that mother now? It depends upon what area you are working in. Forty percent of our mothers did not read or write English in Texas. Spanish was their native tongue, but no educational programs are directed in Spanish. How can you reach that mother? There are two potential channels. You utilize the schools through the PTA. I know of no place where people do not have a school. I know of many places where they do not have a health center. I do not know of a place where the mother cannot get to the store.

I have another pet peeve. The people who have really been shunned are those on the Indian reservations. They may require a different approach; however, food market centers are gradually being expanded on Indian reservations.

Food Markets as a Chance for Education

How do we get through this door? Let me use the problem of goiter as an example. Forty percent of the local groceries in Texas did not stock iodized salt. I suppose from their standpoint, for a good reason. They did know why they should, and they said people never asked for it. In Texas iodized salt does not cost more than uniodized salt. In fact, after my testimony I got a real quick reply from the salt institutions. The manufacturers *do not charge one cent more for iodized salt,* but some retailers do. This is the group we must work with.

We must make a sincere effort to help guide and educate that mother on the best buys, the key foods. For example, I would like to see a sign above the milk chest saying: "This is the milk for preschool children, the one which has Vitamins A and D in it."

Food and Drug indicated to me that this may not be legal, but there
are ways to make it legal. I would like to see it *illegal* to use the
word "imitation milk" on a product. Make them stop using the
word "milk" unless they adequately demonstrate, from a nutritional,
physiological viewpoint that the product is equal to milk. There
are educational approaches through the food industry, the retailer,
and the mother.

I made some statements in our testimony to Congress that there
is less enriched flour used today than there was twenty years ago.
The industry says: "You are not right, you are wrong. Fifty-four
percent of our flour is now enriched and 6 years ago only 50.1
percent was." The World Food War Act Number One of 1941,
made it mandatory to enrich all flour. That was repealed in 1946,
primarily due to the military buying food for 12 million soldiers,
and 90 percent of all flour was enriched. I am not interested in what
was happening in 1955 or 1965. The point is that a good share
of the pre-processed bakery goods are not enriched, and to me that
says you are eating flour which is unenriched. Why not enrich all
flour at the mill? Eight years ago we managed to secure an order
that all overseas shipments of flour be enriched.

A similar problem is that of skimmed milk. USDA is currently
distributing skimmed milk through the commodity distribution program with added Vitamins A and D. If you buy skimmed milk
on the market today with food stamps, it does not have these vitamins
added. I am confident that the milk industry is ready and willing
to push for high standards. I would like to see the nutrition community get out and say that milk is the best food for preschool
children. By that, I mean full-fat milk. I am not a champion for
skimmed milk for preschool children, infants, and weaning children
because I still think that whole milk is the best food.

I think it is ridiculous that Congress, or actually the Administration, was trying to eliminate the School Milk Act. I would not
eliminate it; I would change it to make milk available to every school
age and preschool child. We could do it and we would not have
surplus milk to worry about. I know that there is a small percentage
of children who cannot drink cow's milk. But that is a small percentage, and they become individual problems.

I want to indicate that in this kind of study, there is a whole field opening up for research needs. There are many things in the field of nutritional health that we are not assessing. Some examples are Vitamins B₆, B₁₂, E, trace minerals, fatty acids, amino acids, toxic heavy metals, etc. Why? The answer lies in insufficient funds. We are not assessing some because we do not know enough about them — trace minerals (zinc, chromium, and selenium). These minerals are required by animals. What makes you think that man is so different? You also know that some of these are toxic at certain levels, that they are bound and non-utilizable if one does not have the right mixture.

There are thousands of problems which still require research and knowledge. We do not know enough about some of the problems; however, this does not mean that we should wait for more data before action is taken. We must make sure that children are not growth-retarded from a nutritional standpoint. In our studies we found 18 percent of our mothers who either ate clay, paper or starch. I would not have believed this; in fact, I never heard of paper-eating before. Clay and starch serve as pretty good filtration systems. Is this a social or anthropological problem? Geophasia is very common in Egypt, Iran and the Near East. This is a cause of dwarfism related to zinc deficiency. I am not sure what effect this has on U.S. mothers we have studied. How do we stop it? How do we convince them that they should not do it?

There are some real research problems in terms of how to educate the mother. We tried this procedure: we did a baseline study one year; two years later we went back, and we have had a health impact in that community. So many times, in the field of biochemistry we forget that research is not just restricted to biochemistry. There is research needed on techniques and procedures. I hope that the nutrition community can come up with protocols and ideas and demonstrations. Once you can show a procedure is effective you can market it. I hope we can market nutrition.

DISCUSSION

QUESTIONS TO DR. SCHAEFER

QUESTION: Dr. Schaefer, you stated that the Department of Agriculture says it takes about 75 cents a day to feed a family. I have just returned from working in one of our more liberal states in terms of welfare allowances. The maximum they allow is 63 cents a day. In welfare programs, it ranges from 30 cents to 63 cents, and if you look at statistics you will find an equal number of poverty people not receiving welfare. So we have a high percentage getting way below 75 cents per day for food. This is why I am pushing adequate incomes. For example, in this same state where they are getting 63 cents per day, a family of twelve received $60 a month for rent, $30 a month for heat and utilities, $9 a month for household maintenance, and $30 a month for twelve for clothes. You know what gives, the food budget. So they are using even less. I object to not giving more emphasis to finding what money these families do have for food. My question to you is, when are you going to starting publishing your socio-economic data as it correlates to all of these other findings you have?

ANSWER: I am not going to apologize for not publishing the data. I think if you were in my office and realized the handicaps under which we operate you would more clearly understand. When we started the survey, which was a mandate by Congress, HEW gave us $400,000 to cover two states. We did not receive that money until three or four months after the mandate had gone into effect. We did not receive one cent to do the computer analysis. That was July 1, 1968. We then received all sorts of promises from OEO and everybody else as to assistance in computer help. We now wind up with three separate systems, and it was not until our testimony in January 1969 before the Senate, in which I was asked the question whether we had sufficient funds and facilities to handle the data, that we received verbal support.

I am not apologizing but indicating that we finally, I think, have the procedure worked out now where we will have one computer system. We are analyzing our first two states. You must realize that we have over 200 cards on each individual, something like 200,000 IBM cards that must be edited per state.

We will soon have the report on the first five states which will include social and economic data. In fact, all our data will be presented on the basis of the poverty index gradation. It will list the percent of people who are on welfare and/or food commodities and food stamps in relation to all the parameters we have measured. Our big job will be trying to abstract a few tables that will make sense.

I am glad you made the comment. I did not dwell on the welfare or poverty aspects because I assumed most people knew where I stood on this. You cannot say it is all education or it is all lack of money. I have found from firsthand experience that if I said it was education there is one senator from Louisiana who would say, "We've already taken care of that." When you have families who are really in the poverty area, they need funds. What I say is that funds alone will not solve the whole problem. I am always caught between the facts. Would I rather feed ten children well or feed one hundred with a sprinkle? As I look at some of the programs now, it is like flying over with a jet, opening a bag of flour, letting a little flour hit the poverty groups and saying, "I fed them."

If you look at the statistics the federal bureaucracy presents, you assume they are feeding 7 million. They are not even touching 7 million. They include in some of those statistics kids that go to a day care center one week, or to a camp two weeks a year. They are part of the statistics now. When you talk before a congressman, really all he is interested in is statistics numbers, and dollars. Until we can show them that it is a health problem, and that the programs which are currently involved are not responsive to the needs, we will gain little support.

Now does that mean that you ought to triple or quadruple the food stamp program? I think it is ridiculous to have a price requirement on a food stamp if it is really intended to help the poor. You could probably give less stamps if they had presented evidence of having an income. We have had enough experience to date to indicate that families who cannot get 50 cents together are the real needy.

I agree with your point that 63 cents is allowed and at the same time we say 75 cents is the least cost diet. That is, provided they know how to plan and judiciously buy a proper diet. It gets back to whether or not the U.S. is willing to establish a real welfare system designed with the hope that we will help people off welfare. I am reasonably sure that the teenage mother and her children will have a fair start in the world. They will have that individualism that was talked about yesterday and get out and make a living and not have to be on welfare. But in the meantime we have the poor adults who are trapped and who do need help. It does no good to talk about big fancy federal programs unless they are implemented at the local level.

QUESTION: I think most of us agree with you about the need for milk in the diet. How should we as nutritionists react to the number of physicians who are recommending that the child have either skimmed milk or very little milk in his diet? I do not know whether or not all of you are aware of the fact that there is a movement under way to supply only skimmed milk to school lunches.

ANSWER: That is the time I am ready to take to the street and start carrying a banner. There is plenty of scientific data to prove that a child needs calories, and he needs them from any source he can get them — fats, carbohydrates and protein. You cannot raise a child on corn or wheat which is like skimmed milk to me. You need a fairly concentrated energy source. I certainly would buck the skimmed milk idea. Especially for the preschool child, I support full-fat milk fortified with Vitamin D.

QUESTION: You talked about some money relevant to nutrition education programs. I'd like to find out where that money can come from and where we might find it.

ANSWER: For the first time the HEW administration has testified before Congress that $35 million would be made available to the Department of Education for nutrition education. We were able to obtain $20,000 last year to support a study in Texas where the state Department of Education was calling in seven or eight study groups to review not just nutrition but nutrition, dentistry,immunizations and health activity and to determine how they could update curricula, utilize the school to communicate to the community and to deliver service. I think now it behooves you and others to make sure that the best use is made of the $35 million.

QUESTION: What is the source of this film in Texas? Where can it be purchased or borrowed and what is the name of it?

ANSWER: This is part of our follow-up activities. We are in the process of negotiating for two films. The film is not ready yet. One will depict problems of malnutrition in the teenage pregnant girls by following them all the way through delivery, pointing out both the pros and the cons of their dietary intake. The other would be on the infant.

QUESTION: I am from Indian Health in Billings, and I was not there at the time you did your survey. I reacted to your statement that your study of the Blackfeet was disregarded. Would you please comment?

ANSWER: I meant that it was disregarded at the Washington Public Health Service level. There was really no support given to initiating or taking a look at the food commodity distribution program. I had the privilege of being on the survey of the Blackfeet Indians besides helping support it. What I really meant was that nobody in the higher echelon listened to the fact that there were problems of malnutrition identified in 1961 and that there were problems of ineffective commodity distribution programs on the Indian reservation.

QUESTION: We have $35 million earmarked for nutrition education and I have a big fight with the people who determine what nutrition education is going on in the country. If you are ineffective in getting money and manpower to support the leadership, the nutritionists, where do we go?

ANSWER: We need support for teaching teachers. This means we must train public health nutritionists, or dietitians, or home economists that are majoring in nutrition to really support this battery of people so they in turn can then support the teaching of the field workers. As I look at it, the field workers do not need a Ph.D. A person motivated in the field of social direction with a background in nutrition who could come and get the technical or other information necessary, could work with the local food aides. Agriculture, as you know, has employed something like 5600 food aides, and that is to be expanded to around 10,000. Well, I am disgusted with Public Health. We say we need 100, we said we needed 1,000 back in 1966 to get started, but we have not won that battle yet. Some of the money is needed to support teaching, and I cannot divorce teaching from research, extension, and service. I think these three things go hand in hand.

QUESTION: It seems to me that we are very poor politicians as nutritionists. Doctors also are, and one of my big plugs is to try to get Health and Agriculture together not only on the federal level but also on the state and local levels. This seems to be almost impossible because of the political implications, and I think you brought those out very well. I heard Secretary Harden's testimony and I was shocked to think that we can just earmark money for people and call them aides and yet expect them to do a job when there is so little direction.

ANSWER: You have no argument from me. I will come to Secretary Harden's defense only insofar as this. He inherited the program, and once a program is started in the federal bureaucracy, you cannot shut it off, even if it is ineffecitve. We are saying that what is needed at the state level is to make sure that the trained people in the health and nutrition area make every effort to work with the food aide programs, because the food aide program is here to stay, at least for a while. I thoroughly agree that you cannot legislate this. It will have to be done at the state and local levels. But people are needed. There are 54 state and territorial nutritionists and very few of them have any funds or additional people on their staffs. I am still convinced that we can motivate a lot of people in the American Dietetics Association who are retired or working part time. Also, if you could motivate students to go into this area, you could start making an impact. But without funds and the permission of developing programs at the state level, we are not going to get there.

QUESTION: I would like to say one thing in defense of the nutrition prorgam that has been set up by the Agriculture Department under the Extension Service. That is, never have I seen a program go as far or be as nutritionally sound with less money spent by professional people. Under that particular program, there are professionally trained people from the college on down through the specialists who are definitely nutritionally trained who go from there to county levels to home agents, who are just as specifically and soundly trained, who in turn are training program assistants and reaching those people with sound nutrition from the college level on down. Every bit of that money is used for program assistants and all the professionally trained people are not being given extra money but add this extra load. I will admit we need help, but I still say that we end up with about 24 hours a day that nutrition education is given on a sound basis through the program assistants. I have visited 23 of these low-income families who are the lowest of all low-fed and poorly fed, and I have seen outstanding results from an educational program which is nutritionally sound.

ANSWER: I hope I did not give the impression that the food aide program was ineffective. I have seen some states where we have worked in which they have implemented the program, and I am not saying they are not effective to a certain extent. The fact that these people who have been recruited are out looking for poorer families and identifying them and trying to bring them in to the current available systems — that is essential. I can assure you that in some of the states there is little supervision of training. If you have the competency in the state and you have the motivation where people will be willing to work 24 hours a day, then obviously you are going to make sure that the best is done, and they can do a good job.

I am not disagreeing with you in Colorado and some of the other states that I have not seen. I have seen some states where there is a real need for more technical help. I have maintained from the public health standpoint that the largest resource of people to reach people is through our Extension Program in the Department of Agriculture. According to USDA, there is a county agent in every county and there is a home economics agent in every county. But, how many nutritionists in the Public Health Service do we have? These you can name on your hands.

NEW DIMENSIONS

LINNEA ANDERSON, M.P.H.
Associate Professor
Medical Dietetic Division
Ohio State University
Columbus, Ohio

Introduction

This week we have been offered a wealth of information. As Dr. Dupont made numerous announcements about reporting attendance at these sessions for ADA continuing education credits, I am sure that this group was aware that filing for credit as a registered dietitian implies that each one of us will incorporate the information we gained into our practice of dietetics next week. Registration was accepted by the membership of ADA to encourage "high standards of performance of persons practicing in the profession of dietetics."[1]

As I considered my assignment, New Dimensions, it occurred to me that, after all we have heard about cells, tissues, man and society, it would be appropriate for me to offer you a survival kit: a survival kit to use in coping with the knowledge explosion on all fronts — in both the biological and social sciences. In addition, I will make a few comments on new dimensions as I view them and a few comments on the education of the future practitioners of applied nutrition. And I would share with you the fact that I am viewing this week's program as an individual who has been a practitioner of applied nutrition for thirty years. I have worked primarily with the individual either directly, or indirectly as a clinical instructor through students to the individual. My focus has been and will continue to be the individual.

A Survival Kit

On Monday evening Dr. Grace Goldsmith opened this conference with a comprehensive review of the current definitions of nutrition. As a practitioner of applied nurtition, these definitions do not serve me very well. To survive I have had to derive my own. My definition — probably better labeled a generalization is: As a nutritionist I am concerned with a supply of nutrients to society; to the individual; and ultimately to the cell. This generalization can be diagrammed as follows: Society ⇆ the Individual ⇆ the Cell. Over the years whenever I have blocked out one set of arrows: Society ⇎ the Individual ⇆ the Cell, or given more attention to one arrow than another: Society ⇆ the Individual ⇆ the Cell, I have found myself in serious trouble. This idea is the essence of my survival kit or, if you will, my security blanket. I would be remiss if I did not give credit for this idea to Dr. Bender[2] in England.

Lactose and lactase deficiency have been mentioned by a number of the participants — Dr. Herman, Dr. Moore and Dr. Schaefer to mention three. Therefore, I have chosen lactose and lactase deficiency as a model to illustrate how I use my survival kit. I could have chosen protein and calories, ascorbic acid, or any other nutrient discussed this week.

First, I have to know the foods which supply the nutrient; in this case one food, milk. In the past I was concerned with milk as a beverage and its use in food preparation — primarily baked products and desserts. Today, I have to be aware of the increasing use of dry milk solids in convenience foods.

I also have to keep in mind how processing affects food: in this case the lactose content of milk. On Wednesday morning Dr. Herman was asked why buttermilk might be used by some individuals with lactase deficiency who do not tolerate "sweet" milk. I could not readily answer this question myself but, at the noon break I went to the bookstore here in the Student Center and looked at a few of the books in the Dairy Science section. I discovered that some of the cultures used to make buttermilk ferment lactose. Therefore, some buttermilk may have less lactose than "sweet" milk.

At the same time as I am focusing on this particular nutrient, lactose, I must also consider what I am doing to nutrient intake generally when I counsel an individual with a lactase deficiency — protein, calcium, riboflavin and niacin equivalents.

Starting with the cell in my diagram what do I need to keep in mind about the metabolism of lactose? Lactose, a disaccharide, is made up of two hexoses, a molecule of glucose and one of galactose. While there are numerous exogenous and endogenous sources of glucose, lactose is our primary food source of galactose, an essential component of mucopolysaccharides, glycolipids and other body constituents. A review of the intermediary metabolism of hexoses shows that galactose can be synthesized in the cells, and therefore an exogenous source of this molecule is not required: we can restrict or exclude lactose, the source of galactose, from a diet. Also, on Wednesday, Dr. Herman added some new information for me to add in this area. He pointed out that the substrate, lactose, does not induce the synthesis of the jejunal enzyme, lactase.

Now we can turn to the individual who cannot hydrolyze lactose due to a deficiency of lactase. Individual variation has, over the years, never ceased to fascinate me. Individuals with lactase deficiency are no exception. Welch and his co-workers[3] in Oklahoma City have demonstrated individual variation in the subjects they have studied. Gray[4] at Stanford has demonstrated, using peroral biopsy material, that in some individuals there may be a decrease in the amount, not a total lack, of enzyme. With this information, therefore, I can expect to work with individuals who may be unable to tolerate any lactose to those who may tolerate restricted amounts.

The first step in the approach to any individual is a detailed diet history. To me it is the only way I can identify individual variations or as we more commonly say, differences. At this point in time we do not know the prevalence of lactase deficiency in our population. A careful diet history communicated properly to our co-workers, in this case the physician, may give a clue to an individual's problem — for example, his reason for not drinking milk, "It makes me sick." In retrospect, I am aware of the individual who said to me, "I drink buttermilk, 'sweet' milk makes me sick."

I trust this discussion reinforces Dr. Herman's answer Wednesday afternoon to the question, "Does the practicing dietitian need to learn biochemistry?" His answer as you will remember was, "No, you have to know biochemistry." And I would remind you that the molecules in the metabolic cycles of the cell which Dr. Mathias discussed on Tuesday come from food. Food, as Dr. Griffith[5] has said, is a regulator of metabolism.

Moving to society, the third part of my diagram: it has been interesting to note the interplay this week between the social and biological scientists. Both groups have referred to the prevalence of lactase deficiency in certain societies around the world. The social scientists showed that one has to be concerned not only with the social and cultural aspects of a society, but also with their biological make-up. As we work with individuals in our society whose families came to the U.S. from Africa, China, or Southeast Asia, where lactase deficiency appears to be prevalent, we need to keep in mind that they may not be able to drink milk. I was intrigued when Dr. Moore reported that a tribe in East Africa drink a beer made from fermented milk. Might this practice have evolved because of lactase deficiency?

There is one other comment I wish to make about society. As you will remember, the missionaries of the past have come in for some adverse comments — putting dresses on the Gadsup people of New Guinea (Dr. Leininger) and changing the food practices of a group in India (Dr. Moore). Were we, prior to our recognition of the world-wide prevalence of lactase deficiency, somewhat like the missionaries of old with our distribution of dry skim milk? Did we listen when mothers said it made their babies ill?

There is one more component of my survival kit which does not show in the diagram. In the midst of this knowledge explosion I frequently find myself envying my friends who are specialists: the biochemist who studies enzymes in chicken livers; the anthropologist who goes to a small island in the Pacific for the U.S. Government to discover whether the people of this island are culturally more like Guam or Japan; the sociologist whose research tells me that health workers prefer to help individuals of their own social class; the psychiatrist who asks me, "When are dietitians going to plan a little sin in their diets?"; or the educator who asks me, "How many undigested failures can students survive?" As a generalist I realize

I cannot be a specialist. Therefore, rather than envy my friends who are specialists, I "use" them. I make them and their expertise an integral part of my survival kit.

New Dimensions

Due to the limitation in time I can comment only briefly on new dimensions. One is the nutrient composition of food. In the past a knowledge of the content of protein, crude fat, and carbohydrate in food was adequate. The presentations this week have made it obvious that we now need to know the disaccharide composition of the carbohydrate in a variety of foods. We also recognize we need better data on the fatty acid composition of fats and the amino acid composition of protein. We will have this information when we ask for it. Without this information we cannot meet the demands of the future.

At the same time we need to become more familiar with the effect of food technology on the nutrient composition of food. The food market is changing rapidly: I referred previously to one example, the increased use of dry milk solids in convenience foods. I second Dr. Jerome's recommendation that one survey the products on the shelves of our supermarkets.

Another dimension we must come to grips with is our knowledge of biochemistry. Those of us in applied nutrition cannot be biochemists, but, as Harper[6] at Wisconsin has pointed out, the training of nutrition educators must include a sound background in basic science so that they can translate scientific developments into practical application. And, I would add, communicate intelligently with the research worker. For example: we project a very poor image when we label the diet plan used in the treatment of phenylketonuric infants and children "Low Phenylalanine Diet." This diet plan is not "low" (deficient) in phenylalanine, it is a diet restricted in phenylalanine. It is planned to provide the individual child's phenylalanine requirement without an excess. Phenylalanine is an essential amino acid required by the normal child and by the child with phenylketonuria.

The question of the ethics of using humans in depletion-repletion studies was asked of Dr. Baker on Wednesday. In the university community today a committee of one's peers carefully monitors research where humans are used as subjects. I would raise a question of ethics for those of us in applied nutrition today. Are we sure that we are not harming a patient? With the increasing need to maneuver nutrient intake — for example, in the treatment of patients in renal failure or impending hepatic coma — are we sure we are contributing to the patient's comfort, not his discomfort?

A number of this week's speakers have urged those of us in applied nutrition to direct our attention to the first part of the life cycle — infants, children, and women in the child-bearing years. Both Dr. Miller and Dr. Goodman emphasized that the "time is now" to be concerned with the adequacy of nutrient intake of pregnant women and infants. And today, Dr. Schaefer voiced his concern about our nutrition education programs in elementary and secondary schools.

If one looks back in the history of applied nutrition in the United States it will be observed that mothers and their infants and children were the primary focus of nutrition services. In my files is the publication, "Goals for Nutrition Education for Elementary and Secondary Schools," prepared by the Department of Nutrition, Harvard School of Public Health, and distributed by the Nutrition Foundation, Inc. The copyright date is 1947!

Granted recent research on the relationship of nutrient intake to growth of the fetus and infant puts our counseling on a firmer scientific basis but, one is forced to raise the question — why do we need to be urged to *re-direct* our attention to mothers and their children? Have we been prone to conquer new worlds (chronic diseases in adults) at the expense of losing past gains?[7]

In addition to using appropriately the research in the biological sciences we also need to listen to the social scientists. They have been telling us that the nuclear family has replaced the extended family in our society. In interpret this to mean that child-rearing practices are transmitted by health workers today, not by parents and grandparents as in the past. Therefore, each new generation in our society will require our services in nutrition education and counseling. Let us hope that twenty years hence at a conference on Dimensions of Nutrition, we will not be urged to re-direct our attention, rather be urged to continue to sustain our interest in the first part of the life cycle.

Education of the Future Practitioner

The traditional programs which have prepared the practitioner of applied nutrition are changing: more needs to be done. A course in biochemistry is a requirement but, do we help the student to bridge the gap between this and his nutrition courses? One step in this direction is a recent publication, "Determination of Concepts Basic to an Improved Foods and Nutrition Curriculum at the College Level," the work of a project directed by Dr. Dorothy H. Strong at the University of Wisconsin. Three areas are included in the statements of concepts and generalizations: food materials; biological aspects of human nutrition; and human behavior in relation to food.

We also need to look at how we are preparing the future practitioner to function in the clinical setting — to work with people. Coordinated undergraduate programs similar to the one we have at Ohio State University is one approach. More innovation in our educational programs which put the future practicioner into the counseling role as a student should be emerging.

And, finally, as the young, bright-eyed activist graduates from college today, one hopes her ideas meet with acceptance; that she can explore and try new ideas and does not have her enthusiasm dampened by, "but we have always done it this way."

One final comment: as I have listened this week to the biochemist, molecular biologist, physician and anthropologist, and to the informal conversation of the group, it has occurred to me that the "time is now" for us to re-read Caroline Hunt's biography* of Ellen Richards, one of the founders of the Home Economics movement. Mrs. Richards began her career in the 1870's as a chemist at the Massachusetts Institute of Technology and in the 1890's and early 1900's moved out into the community to work to improve the conditions of the poor in Boston, particularly problems in foods and nutrition.

As a self-appointed committee of one, I wish to express for those in attendance at this conference our appreciation to the Colorado Dietetic Association; the committee which planned the program; and to Dr. Dupont and the faculty of Colorado State University, who gave so generously of their time and expertise.

---

*Published by the American Home Economics Association, 1935.

REFERENCES

1. *ADA Courier.* June, 1969.

2. Bender, Arnold. "The Nutritionist in Industry," in *Changing Food Habits.* Yudkin, J. and J. C. McKenzie, eds. MacGibbon and Kee (London, 1964).

3. Welsh, J. D., et al. Studies of Lactose Intolerance in Families, *Arch. Intern. Med.,* 122:315, 1968.

4. Gray, G. M. Persistent Deficiency of Intestinal Lactase in Apparently Cured Tropical Sprue, *Gastroenterology,* 54:552, 1968.

5. Griffith, W. H. Food as a Regulator of Metabolism, *Am. Jour. Clin. Nutr.,* 17:391, 1965.

6. Harper, A. E. Nutrition: Where Are We? Where Are We Going? *Am. Jour. Clin. Nutr.,* 22:87, 1969.

7. Anderson, L. and J. H. Browe. *Nutrition and Family Health Services* W. B. Saunders Co. (Philadelphia, 1960), p. 3.